HEALTH BY THE PEOPLE

HEALTH
BY THE PEOPLE

Edited by

KENNETH W. NEWELL

Director,
Division of Strengthening of Health Services,
World Health Organization,
Geneva, Switzerland

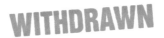

WORLD HEALTH ORGANIZATION

GENEVA

1975

1st Impression 1975

2nd Impression 1977

ISBN 92 4 156042 8

PRINTED IN SWITZERLAND

CONTENTS

FOREWORD

The condition of the rural majority of the population of the developing world has been presented many times in economic, organizational, and health terms. Nearly all accounts are gloomy and some describe both the present state and the speed of change in a way that makes us doubt the acceptability or the effectiveness of solutions. But our view must depend upon what we hear and sometimes it is difficult to listen to, and to understand, all of the voices.

In this book a group of persons close to the villagers themselves from many different countries have gathered to give us their examples of possible health solutions. The scale of their examples ranges from the country to the village and their outlook has been properly conditioned by both the good and the bad experiences they have passed through.

I consider that within this diversity of experience and outlook there are some common messages and qualities in addition to the pleas for help. We should listen to these voices and add to our own knowledge and then consider whether their conclusions could influence our attitudes and actions.

Director-General

INTRODUCTION

KENNETH W. NEWELL [a]

There is little doubt that a visitor from another world looking down upon the earth would find much to be puzzled about. He would see as much as 80% of the world's population spread within a lush green area sandwiched between the concentrated dark blobs of the cities and the grey browns of the deserts and mountains. It would be natural for him to assume that these rural people were the primary strength of the human race and were particularly favoured. However, as he came nearer he would observe that most of them were physically confined to a small plot of land and socially tied to a group as small as an extended family or clan. Rather than order or organization, he would see drought-stricken areas side by side with flooded areas, dry fields beside rivers taking water to the sea, and persons sitting or waiting, apparently powerless as disaster inevitably approaches. The possibility that there would be economic, ecological, nutritional disaster, disease and death would appear to be self-evident, and yet the people would appear to sit with blank faces apparently unaware that a hundred, a thousand, or a million pairs of hands working together could influence their future and stave off the disaster to come.

Great changes for the better have occurred during this century. We must recognize these achievements, but while we do so we must also be perceptive enough to understand to what point these victories have taken us. The majority of the rural populations of the world do not have sufficient food to enable them to have a normal growth and development; one out of four of the children of many groups dies before the age of one year; epidemic and endemic communicable diseases are a day-to-day reality; and maybe 80% of these people have little or no contact at all with what we call health technology, which is so often quoted as a shining example of present-day man's technological ingenuity and progress.

The lot of many rural populations has improved even when viewed through the doubting eyes of a health worker. However, their present state is sufficiently well documented for us to have few doubts that the

---

[a] Director, Division of Strengthening of Health Services, World Health Organization, Geneva, Switzerland.

point we have reached is still intolerable. We have no overall indicator of rural hopelessness. Even those fragments of "fact" that we call health statistics are all too often incomplete and inaccurate. This is not surprising when we consider that the efforts involved in their collection must compete against other imperatives and that they are often unwelcome if they mainly document failure or shame. Despite the improvements that have taken place, the ground-level view is still one of swollen-bellied children playing in the dust of the village square, of lines of women carrying water, and of the scratching of little patches of land with a stick as the desert creeps nearer.

It is very easy to throw up one's hands or to shut one's eyes to these sights and sounds. If one uses the most simple arithmetic to add up all that is needed to counter the worst of the evils, it would appear that there will never be enough resources. There appears to be no starting-point, no proper way to start. The step from hopelessness to hope may appear too big for us to consider in a time scale of less than a century. Some people say that such a conclusion is not that of a pessimist but that of a realist. Other people do not agree. Such sums and such thinking, they hold, are products of our own way of looking at the world. They ignore a whole series of factors and strengths that we cannot and should not quantify and put into an equation. They ignore what has been done and is being done in various parts of the world. A different conclusion is possible.

This book is about rural populations, but its main emphasis is upon health and health services. The relationship between rural hopelessness and health is a complex one. Ill health adds to hopelessness, but its removal does not mean that there is hope. We can describe endemic or epidemic diseases, stunted children, deaths occurring mostly in infancy and childhood, no help in an emergency, maternal deaths against such a background as we have indicated; but the background and the description would have to be different if the people were healthy and strong. We should have to add such qualities as hope, human dignity, a capacity for improvement and change, organization and responsibility, and mastery over one's own fate. The problem and the priority have to be the total rural hopelessness complex and not just ill health. We are only slowly beginning to understand that people themselves are aware that health may have a low ranking among the starting points for change.

It is difficult to work out the reasons why members of the health services have tried to separate "health concerns" from other parts of the complex. Is it because we do not understand the problem or feel incompetent or powerless to influence the main issues, or because we want to "control" our own field? Whatever the reason, it is clearly not because we have scientific "evidence" that it is the most effective or the cheapest way or that it is what the people want. On the contrary, we have studies demonstrating that many of the "causes" of common health problems derive from parts of society itself and that a strict health sectoral approach is ineffective, other actions outside the field of health perhaps having greater health effects than strictly health interventions. If we do not consider our restricted approach to be valid, then our reaction to its rejection is even more strange. As the health services fail in their bid for additional resources to further their priorities, the health professions turn their backs on the problem and direct their energies towards developing additional methods for helping the privileged people who can both afford and appreciate them.

Such views could be said to be widely held, but they also are biased as they ignore some events that have been taking place during the past 25 years. Individual groups and some states have tried to approach the problem from a different direction. Some have tried to extend services, including health, outwards towards the villages. Some countries have tried to face the total problem by an interlocking series of political, economic, and social measures. Some individuals have tried to build upwards and outwards with the villagers, using health benefits as trigger mechanisms or consequential benefits of change. Health workers and health service techniques have frequently played an important role in these endeavours.

All of us who have seen or heard about the results of these endeavours want to know more. We feel that we may have missed something that could be important. We want to have more than purely "before and after" data. We want to find out what really happened and why this effort was a success in one place while it was a failure somewhere else. We rarely receive a useful answer.

For this reason WHO, as an extension of a joint WHO/UNICEF study in 1974, decided to ask a group of people who participated in some of these attempts at change to write down what happened. While some data were necessary to put the changes into a meaningful perspective, the authors were asked to give especial prominence to the process itself. What was wanted was a series of stories that would give life and colour to the sequence of events and decisions they considered important. This was a difficult or impossible request. Active participants are not always good story tellers. No single individual is fully responsible for a national change and he may feel diffident about giving a personal view. Many projects or programmes were still a long way from reaching even their intermediate goals.

An added difficulty was that as one looked for examples one found more than could be included in a single volume, so that some have had to be omitted. This book is, therefore, a selection of examples from many different countries and includes areas as large as China and as small as a Guatemalan Indian village. It has contributions from observers (China), from national participants (Cuba, Tanzania, Venezuela), from local groups (India, Indonesia, Iran), and from persons who participated (Guatemala, Niger). Many of the authors have had the collaboration of WHO staff members who have observed their projects or programmes and have assisted in preparing their section for publication. As editor I have selected the examples given and regret having had to exclude others for reasons of space.

The criteria for selection have not been dependent on WHO sponsorship or involvement; WHO has played little or no direct part in many of the programmes chosen. I have not attempted to correct or change any of the contributions except for purposes of clarity. Responsibility for the accuracy, balance, and conclusions of each contribution rests exclusively with the authors concerned. The accounts are given in the authors' own words and it is hoped that the differences in approach and style will be seen as a refreshing expression of the diversity of the endeavours throughout the world.

WHO has two motives in publishing this book. One is to present once again the problems that the world has to face; the other is to present successful solutions to them, in the hope that information about existing successes will encourage others to seek out new paths. There appear to be many roads to success. Indeed, if there is a moral to this book it is that possibilities for change are open to all people but no standard method is applicable to them all.

THE HEALTH CARE DELIVERY SYSTEM OF THE PEOPLE'S REPUBLIC OF CHINA

VICTOR W. SIDEL & RUTH SIDEL

There is common agreement that prior to 1949 the state of health of large numbers of the Chinese people was extremely poor and that the health services provided for them were grossly inadequate. The people of China in the 1930s and 1940s suffered from the consequences of widespread poverty, poor sanitation, continuing war, and rampant disease. The crude death rate was estimated at about 25 deaths per 1000, one of the world's highest death rates. The infant mortality rate was about 200 per 1000 live births; in other words, one out of every 5 babies born died in its first year of life (1). Most deaths in China were due to infectious diseases, usually complicated by some form of malnutrition. Prevalent infectious diseases included bacterial illnesses such as cholera, diphtheria, gonorrhoea, leprosy, meningococcal meningitis, plague, relapsing fever, syphilis, tetanus, tuberculosis, typhoid fever, and typhus; viral illnesses such as Japanese B encephalitis, smallpox, and trachoma; and parasitic illnesses such as ancylostostomiasis (hookworm disease), clonorchiasis, filariasis, kala-azar, malaria, paragonimiasis, and schistosomiasis (2).

A picture of health in Shanghai, one of the most industrialized cities in China, was given by a Canadian hotel manager who returned to China in 1965 and sought the sights he had known for the twenty years prior to 1949.

I searched for scurvy-headed children. Lice-ridden children. Children with inflamed red eyes. Children with bleeding gums. Children with distended stomachs and spindly arms and legs. I searched the sidewalks day and night for children who had been purposely deformed by beggars. Beggars who would leech on to any well-dressed passer-by to black-mail sympathy and offering, by pretending the hideous-looking child was their own.

I looked for children covered with horrible sores upon which flies feasted. I looked for children having a bowel movement, which, after much strain, would only eject tapeworms.

I looked for child slaves in alleyway factories. Children who worked twelve hours a day, literally chained to small press punches. Children who, if they lost a finger, or worse, often were cast into the streets to beg and forage in garbage bins for future subsistence (3).

Preventive medicine was almost non-existent in most of China except for areas where special projects were conducted, usually with foreign funding. Therapeutic medicine of the modern scientific type (which the

1

Chinese call *xiyi* or "Western medicine") was almost completely unavailable in the rural areas—where 80% of China's people live—and for most poor urban dwellers. Estimates of the number of physicians in China in 1949 who were trained in Western medicine vary from 10 000 to 40 000 (*4*); the best estimate seems to be about 20 000, or approximately one doctor for every 25 000 of the roughly 500 million population of China at that time. Most of these were either doctors from Western countries, usually missionaries, or doctors trained in schools supported and directed from abroad; they were mainly concentrated in the cities of eastern China. Nurses and other types of health workers were in even shorter supply. The maximum estimate of the number of hospital beds in 1949 was 90 000, or less than one bed per 5000 people.

There had been some very localized efforts in the 1930s to train new types of health worker to meet the needs of China's rural population, but these efforts also were largely supported from abroad and usually poorly supported by the people they were supposed to serve and poorly integrated with their life and needs.

The bulk of the medical care available to the Chinese people was provided by the roughly half million practitioners of traditional medicine (*zhongyi* or "Chinese medicine"), who ranged from poorly educated pill peddlers to well-trained and widely experienced practitioners of the medicine the Chinese had developed over two millenia. These practitioners and those who practised Western medicine were deeply mistrustful of each other and blocked each others' efforts in many ways.

Probably most important of all, three-fourths of the Chinese people were said to be illiterate. Cycles of flood and drought kept most of the people starving or at the least undernourished. And the limited resources that did exist were maldistributed, so that a few lived in comfort and the vast majority lived a life of grinding poverty. Feelings of powerlessness and hopelessness were widespread; individual efforts were of little avail and community efforts were almost impossible to organize.

Experiments in meeting these needs were started during the 1930s and 1940s by Mao Tse-tung and the People's Liberation Army that he led, first in Kiangsi Province and then, after the Long March, in the areas around Yenan in Shensi Province. These efforts involved mobilizing the people to educate themselves and encouraging them individually and collectively to provide their own health care and medical care services.

With the assumption of state power by Mao and the Chinese Communist Party in 1949 (which the Chinese call the "Liberation") this experience was expanded into a national policy, which included the following elements:

(1) Medicine should serve the needs of the workers, peasants, and soldiers—that is, those who previously had the least services were now to be the specially favoured recipients of services.

2

(2) Preventive medicine should be put first—that is, where resources were limited, preventive medicine was to take precedence over therapeutic medicine.

(3) Chinese traditional medicine should be integrated with Western scientific medicine—that is, instead of competing, the practitioners of the two types of medical care should learn from each other.

(4) Health work should be conducted with mass participation—that is, everyone in the society was to be encouraged to play an organized role in the protection of his own health and that of his neighbours.

Some of the efforts of the 1950s and early 1960s were based on models from other countries, particularly the Soviet Union, which provided a large amount of technical assistance to China during this period. A number of new medical schools were established, some of the older ones were moved from the cities of the east coast to areas of even greater need further west, and class size was vastly expanded. "Higher" medical education usually consisted of 6 years, following the completion of some 12 years of previous education, although some schools accepted students with less previous schooling and some were said to graduate them after only 4 or 5 years of medical education. One school, the China Medical College located in the buildings of the former Peking Union Medical College, had an 8-year curriculum and was devoted to the training of teachers and researchers. These efforts produced a remarkably large number of "higher" medical graduates, including stomatologists, pharmacologists, and public health specialists as well as physicians. It has been estimated that more than 100 000 doctors were trained over 15 years, an increase of some 500% (4). But by 1965 China's population had increased to about 700 million, and the doctor/population ratio was still less than one per 5000 people.

At the same time large numbers of "middle" medical schools were established to train assistant doctors (modelled in some ways on the Soviet feldshers), nurses, midwives, pharmacists, technicians, and sanitarians. These schools accepted students after 9 or 10 years of schooling and had a curriculum of 2 to 3 years. It has been estimated that some 170 000 assistant doctors, 185 000 nurses, 40 000 midwives, and 100 000 dispensers were trained (4).

In addition to these efforts to produce rapidly many more professional health workers, people in the community were mobilized to perform health-related tasks themselves. A large-scale attack was made on illiteracy and superstition. By means of mass campaigns, people were organized so as to accomplish together what they could not do individually. One of the best known of these campaigns (which were often called the Great Patriotic Health Campaigns) was the one aimed at eliminating the "four

3

pests", originally identified as flies, mosquitos, rats and grain-eating sparrows; when the elimination of sparrows appeared likely to produce serious ecological problems, bedbugs (and in some areas lice or cockroaches) were substituted (5). People were also encouraged to build sanitation facilities and to keep their neighbourhoods clean.

Campaigns against specific diseases were also mounted. Thousands of people were trained in short courses to recognize the symptoms and signs of venereal disease, to encourage treatment, and to administer antibiotics when necessary; at the same time the brothels were closed and the prostitutes were treated and retrained (6). There were also mass campaigns against opium use. Epidemic prevention centres were established to conduct massive immunization campaigns and to educate people in sanitation and other prevention techniques.

The classic example of the use of mass organization in health was the campaign against schistosomiasis. This campaign was based, according to J. S. Horn (7), on the concept of the "mass line"—"the conviction that the ordinary people possess great strength and wisdom and that when their initiative is given full play they can accomplish miracles." Before the peasants were organized to fight against the snails, they were thoroughly educated in the nature of schistosomiasis by means of lectures, films, posters, and radio talks. They were then mobilized twice a year, in March and August, and, together with voluntary labour from the People's Liberation Army, students, teachers, and office workers, they drained the rivers and ditches, buried the banks of the rivers, and smoothed down the buried dirt. The idea behind the antischistosomiasis programme was not only to recruit the people to do the work but also to mobilize their enthusiasm and initiative so that they would fight the disease (7).

The antischistosomiasis effort is particularly revealing, since it mobilized the population in several directions: to move against the snails, to cooperate in case-finding and treatment, and to improve environmental sanitation. Yukiang County in Kiangsi Province, for example, had been plagued by schistosomiasis for more than 100 years. According to one report (8), 1 million m² of land was infested with snails, and the "average" infection rate among the peasants was 21.4%. After investigating the prevalence of the disease, the antischistosomiasis station was set up in the county in 1953. When the campaign started, the personnel of the station began publicizing its purposes, as well as health work in general, using

broadcasting, wall newspapers, blackboards, exhibits of real and model objects, lantern-slide shows, and dramatic performances. Related scientific knowledge was also popularized. To help the peasants raise their political consciousness, break their superstitious belief in gods, devils, and fate, and to build up their confidence in conquering the disease, meetings were organized for recalling sufferings in the old society and comparing them with the happiness in the new society. Through these activities the confidence of the broad mass in the certain triumph of their struggle against schistosomiasis was gradually built up and further strengthened.

4

Once the population learned about schistosomiasis, a "people's war" was launched against the snails. From 1955 to 1957, 20 000 peasants in Yukiang County filled up old ditches and ponds, dug new ditches, and expanded the cultivation area by roughly 90 acres (36 ha). Special methods had to be used in some areas. For example, three lotus ponds, each 3 feet (1 m) deep, covering several acres contained snails in high density that people had attempted to exterminate by removing the surface soil, burning aquatic vegetation, and other methods, but the snails had not been completely eliminated. Finally the ponds were drained, all grass and vegetation at the bottom were burned, and snail-free mud was piled on top and pounded so that the snails were suffocated. Seven square or rectangular fish ponds were then created out of the three former snail-breeding ponds.

After this massive war on schistosomiasis, however, it was still necessary to check for the recurrence of snails, as well as on water control and waste disposal, so the people had to be educated in the treatment of human excreta, the provision of safe drinking-water, and improved personal hygiene. Production teams under the leadership of health workers are responsible for these public health measures.

Health work in Heilungkiang Province in the north-east was described in an article in *China's Medicine* in 1968 (9). In order to promote health education in the province, mass meetings were called in 60 cities and counties, leaflets and pamphlets on health were distributed, and students began to engage in health education among the workers and peasants. It was estimated that in two counties 250 000 middle and primary school students were mobilized for this work. Needless to say, the students learned as much as they taught.

In all these health campaigns it was repeatedly stressed that health is important not only for the individual's wellbeing but also for that of the family, the community, and the country as a whole. The basic concept is said to be the recognition of a problem important to large numbers of people, the analysis of the problem and recommendation of solutions by technical and political leaders, and then—most important—the thorough discussion of the analysis and recommended solutions with the people so that they can fully accept them as their own. Using the techniques of mobilizing the general population to participate actively in the provision of medical care and the prevention of illness, diseases such as smallpox, cholera, typhoid fever, and plague were completely eliminated. Venereal disease and kala-azar were practically eliminated, and diseases such as malaria and filariasis are being rapidly brought under control. Tuberculosis, trachoma, schistosomiasis, and ancylostomiasis are still not under full control although their prevalence is being markedly reduced (2). In short, the successes in the prevention of infectious disease over a time-span of only one generation were truly monumental.

In therapeutic medicine, the campaign to integrate Chinese medicine with Western medicine was designed (1) to make full use of those elements of Chinese medicine that were found effective; (2) to provide greater acceptance of Western techniques among those, particularly in the rural areas, who mistrusted them; and (3) to employ efficiently the large numbers of practitioners of Chinese medicine. The campaign met with some success but there was still said to be considerable resistance on both sides. Perhaps of even greater importance, there was said still to be considerable resistance on the part of "higher" medical graduates to practising in the rural areas where there was the greatest need for them. As a result much of the large rural population still lacked adequate access to medical care.

In 1965, in one of the forerunners of what came to be known as the Great Proletarian Cultural Revolution, Mao severely criticized the Ministry of Health for what he called its over-attention to urban problems. He urged a series of changes in medical education, medical research, and medical practice. His statement, known throughout China as the June 26th Directive, concluded: "In medical and health work, put the stress on the rural areas!" As a result of this directive, and of the Cultural Revolution of 1966–1969 itself, much in medicine was markedly reorganized. Higher medical schools began again to admit students who had less previous schooling but had experience of working in factories and in communes; these students were usually selected by the people with whom they had worked and whom they were to return to serve. The curriculum was restructured to place greater emphasis on practical rather than theoretical aspects, with much more training in Chinese medicine, and was experimentally reduced to about 3½ years instead of 6 as previously. Medical research in the institutes of the Chinese Academy of Medical Sciences began to place much greater emphasis on the treatment of common illnesses and especially on the role of techniques of Chinese medicine.

The Cultural Revolution also brought about great changes in medical practice. Previously, some mobile health teams had travelled the countryside providing services and training, but now mobile medical teams were organized on a massive scale. Most urban medical workers were required to play a role in these teams or in other work in the rural areas, and a rotation system was operated so that at any given time about one-third of urban health workers were serving outside the cities. They were there not only to provide services for those living in the countryside but also to be themselves "re-educated" by the experience.

Part of their responsibility was the training of large numbers of peasants to provide environmental sanitation, health education, preventive medicine, first aid, and primary medical care while continuing their farm work. These peasant health workers came to be known as "barefoot doctors" in the rural areas near Shanghai, where much agricultural work is done barefoot in the rice paddies. Although the barefoot doctors wear shoes most of the time, and especially while performing their medical tasks, the term is used to emphasize the fact that these personnel perform their medical work together with their tasks as farm workers.

With regard to environmental sanitation, the barefoot doctor has responsibility, for example, for the proper disposal and later use of human faeces as fertilizer, for the purity of drinking-water, and for the control of and campaigns against "pests". Many of the sanitation tasks are usually carried out by more junior health aides, whom the barefoot doctor trains and supervises. Immunizations are an important responsibility of the barefoot doctor, but these too are often performed by the health aides, who do their work during lunch hours and "spare time".

Health education and the provision of primary medical care are other important tasks of the barefoot doctor. He is also readily available to deal with medical emergencies, since he often works in the fields with his patients and lives among them. He is said to be skilled in first aid and in the treatment of "minor and common illnesses". Perhaps most important, his fellow workers know him well and trust him.

Some idea of the range of what the barefoot doctor is supposed to know is provided by barefoot doctor handbooks, of which a number are now available. The handbooks cover a broad range of medical problems and discuss both traditional Chinese and Western treatment (10). Another, perhaps more direct, measure of what the barefoot doctor does is the drugs he is empowered to use. These range from traditional herb remedies to antibiotics, epinephrine, reserpine, and other powerful modern drugs, but other drugs with great toxic potential, such as digitalis and adrenal corticosteroids, are not generally used by the barefoot doctor. Visitors discussing these items with barefoot doctors have been impressed by their remarkably detailed knowledge of the nature of the medications, the indications and contraindications, and the possible adverse reactions.

The initial training for the barefoot doctors, of whom there are now said to be over a million, usually takes place locally for a period of 3 months, often in the commune hospital or county hospital. Subsequent continuing supervision and training periods are used to improve their knowledge and skills. Barefoot doctors are encouraged to use a wide range of both traditional Chinese and Western medicines and some have become skilled enough to perform limited forms of major surgery. The complex system of supervision and referral appears to ensure that there is adequate control of technical quality as well as rational deployment of manpower and access to services.

China's countryside is divided into communes; these are divided into production brigades, which in turn are divided into production teams. The barefoot doctors usually work in health stations at the production brigade level, but do much of their work, both medical and agricultural, with their fellow members of the production team. The barefoot doctor's income is generally determined in the same way as that of the other peasants in his commune; each peasant's earnings depend on the total income of his brigade and the number of "work points" that he collects. The barefoot doctor earns work points for medical work just as he would for agricultural work. The barefoot doctors are selected by their fellow peasants for training, and these co-workers often choose the most capable barefoot doctor for education as a physician.

There are health workers analogous to the barefoot doctor in the factories (where they are called "worker doctors") and in the urban neighbourhoods. They too are selected by their fellow workers and receive short periods of initial training, usually 1 or 2 months. They provide preventive medicine, health education, occupational health services, first aid, and limited primary care functions on the factory floor or in the factory health centre. A system of supervision, continuing education, and referral is provided through the doctors and assistant doctors in the factory or in the neighbourhood clinic. The worker doctor, like the barefoot doctor, performs health work part-time while continuing his other duties, and is paid a salary similar to that of other workers in the factory.

The cities of China are divided into districts of several hundred thousand people, the districts are divided into "neighbourhoods" or "streets" of about 50 000 people, the neighbourhoods are divided into "residents' committees" or "lanes" of about 5000 people, and the residents' committees into "groups" of about 100 people. Services are decentralized to the lowest level at which they can be given (11). Many social services are provided at the group level by elected group leaders and deputy group leaders. Residents' committees usually have health stations in which the personnel are local housewives or retired people trained for short periods and called "Red Medical Workers". These workers are trained and supervised by the doctors and assistant doctors who work in the clinic or hospital at the neighbourhood level; they can refer patients to those facilities or directly to the district general hospital when necessary.

One of the most important tasks of China's health workers and neighbourhood and commune leaders is felt to be the reduction of China's birth rate. In the urban areas health workers in the lanes and neighbourhoods play an important role in birth control campaigns. Education is one of the most important aspects of the programme and is carried out by means of booklets and other printed materials and, even more important, through residents' committees, Red Medical Workers, and other person-to-person contacts. The emphasis is on the importance of family planning in building a new socialist society rather than on the Malthusian concepts of over-population leading to poverty and famine. Family planning is "based upon the emancipation of the woman, her equality, her right to study and participate in all political decisions, and her heightened social consciousness. Planned parenthood and marriage are factors for the promotion of a socialist society, but they must be based on full equality of both partners, self-respect, and knowledge. It is therefore essential that the masses themselves should grasp all the factors of health work, and themselves carry out the programme." (12)

The Chinese Marriage Law of 1950 provides that women may marry at the age of 18 and men at 20, but a vigorous and successful campaign has been waged to delay the age of marriage. In the cities the age urged for marriage is now said to be 26–29 for men and 24–26 for women. Late marriage is an important method of population control; many mothers are giving birth to their first babies in their late twenties or early thirties. The optimum family size in the cities is now considered to be two or three children, and tubal or vas deferens ligation is often urged after the birth of the second or third child.

In the urban lanes, Red Medical Workers are responsible for the dissemination of birth control information. Health workers go from door to door, talking with the women about the number of children they want and the birth control methods they are using. By means of monthly visits to the home of each woman of "childbearing age", which is defined as the time of marriage to menopause, the Red Medical Workers keep careful track of the contraceptives used. Most of these workers are housewives, often with two or three children; many have had tubal ligations themselves, so they serve as models for the women they visit. It was said that while no one was "forced" to limit the family to two or three children, great stress is put on educating people in the importance—not necessarily to themselves, but rather to the neighbourhood, the city, and the nation—of population control. Abortions are free and easily available but are almost never requested by unmarried women; pregnancies among unmarried women are exceedingly rare and births out of wedlock are practically unknown. Abortion is viewed as a method to be used when birth control fails, not as a primary method of contraception (13).

In the rural areas midwives trained for short periods (usually 6 months) provide birth control information and antenatal and postnatal care, and perform simple deliveries. The midwife has an intimate, person-to-person relationship with the women of the brigade, with emphasis on education and persuasion. The midwife may provide oral contraceptives directly to the woman but the insertion of the intrauterine device and the performing of abortions, tubal ligations, and vas deferens ligations is done in the commune hospital.

There are many factors contributing to the significantly higher birth rate in China's rural areas than in the cities: the traditional need to have many children for a few to survive; the need for sons, who would remain at home upon reaching adulthood and help with the farming, in contrast to daughters, who were obliged to live with their husbands' families and therefore contributed little or no work to their parents' home; the current system of work points by which families with a larger number of workers have a greater income; the fact that children in rural areas must care for elderly parents because of the lack of a pension system such as that which protects retired workers in the urban areas; and a residual "feudal ideology", often expressed by grandmothers, which favours having more children, preferably male children. Chinese health workers are attempting at every level to persuade peasants to think, feel, and act differently with regard to "planned birth" but, although progress is being made, birth rates in the countryside remain higher than in urban areas.

In Shanghai City, which probably has the most effective programme, the crude birth rate in 1972 was reported to be about 7 per 1000; this, combined with its crude death rate of about 6 per 1000, implies a natural growth rate of only 1 per 1000, or 0.1% (14). Other cities appear to have crude birth rates of between 10 and 20 per 1000; that of Peking City, for example, is reported to be 14 per 1000. Many communes have crude birth rates between 15 and 25 per 1000, but communes in outlying and minority group areas are said to have higher rates; indeed, there is no attempt to encourage birth control among the minority group peoples. The overall pattern, however, is a great decline from China's crude birth rate in the 1950s, which is estimated to have been over 40 per 1000.

Other achievements of the Chinese health care system include technical advances such as the treatment of widespread severe burns, the replantation of severed limbs, and—most recently—new uses of techniques derived from traditional Chinese medicine. These have included the employment of acupuncture to produce hypalgesia during surgical procedures, thus avoiding the dangers to certain patients of general anaesthesia, and the study of a number of traditional herbal medicines in an attempt to isolate and identify active extracts and to determine their effectiveness using scientific criteria.

Although statistics are not yet available on the current health status of China's population, recent visitors report a nation of healthy-looking, vigorous people. While it is clear that the nation is still poorly developed technologically and its people—particularly in the rural areas—work very long and hard, there is no evidence of the malnutrition, ubiquitous infectious disease, and other ill-health that often accompanies poverty.

In one city, Shanghai, health statistics are becoming available. They show a crude death rate of 6 per 1000, an infant mortality rate of 9 per 1000 live births (15), and correspondingly low age-specific death rates at other ages. The life expectancy at birth now appears to be about 70 years. The leading causes of death are now reported to be cancer, stroke, and heart disease (16). Shanghai City is certainly not representative of the rest of China, or even of its other large cities, but the remarkable changes over the past two decades in Shanghai—the infant mortality rate in 1948 was estimated at 150 per 1000—are probably indicative of rapid changes in health status throughout China.

These changes in health status are certainly not the result of changes in health care alone; improvements in nutrition, sanitation, and living standards are at least as important. But the changes in health care have certainly played an important role. In summary, the principles used included:

(1) A fundamental redistribution of health care resources from the service of those who formerly had most to those who had least. This is being accomplished, especially since the Cultural Revolution, by means of society's full control over those resources, with little or none remaining in the private sector, and by a shift in emphasis towards narrowing the gap between the urban and rural areas.

(2) A commitment to encouraging the people's own self-reliance and mutual help in meeting health problems. This is being accomplished by mass education, special nationwide campaigns, and intensive local neighbourhood organization, using techniques that emphasize the importance of health for the family, community, and nation rather than merely for individual wellbeing.

(3) The training of a large number of full-time professional health workers. This is being accomplished by vastly expanding existing schools and establishing many new ones and, especially since the Cultural Revolution, by exploring techniques for shortening training. But the number of workers who have been trained—though vast—is still insufficient to meet the needs of China's population.

(4) The training, more recently, of large numbers of part-time health workers who continue at the same time to be peasants, workers, or housewives. This is being accomplished largely through local initiative but with the cooperation of professional health workers in training, supervision, and referral.

(5) An emphasis on preventive rather than therapeutic medicine. This is being accomplished by formulating nationwide policies for sanitation, immunization, and other preventive measures and then mobilizing for their local implementation.

(6) Attempts to preserve and strengthen that which was most valuable in traditional Chinese medicine and using it and its practitioners as a vehicle for the wider distribution of modern medicine. This is being accomplished by bringing together traditional and modern practitioners in their medical practice and by training each type in the others' techniques.

(7) Motivation through fostering a desire for service to others rather than for individual self-aggrandizement. This is being accomplished by widespread campaigns, through every medium of public communication, emphasizing the importance of "serving the people".

REFERENCES

1. Szeming Sze. *China's health problems*, Washington, D.C., Chinese Medical Association, 1943
2. Huang Kun-yen. Infectious and parasitic diseases. In: Quinn, J. R., ed. *Medicine and public health in the People's Republic of China*, Washington, D.C., National Institutes of Health, 1972, pp. 263–288
3. Scott, W. A. China revisited by an old China hand. *Eastern Horizon*, 5 (6): 34–40 (1966)
4. Orleans, L. A. Medical education and manpower in Communist China. In: C. T. Hu, ed. *Aspects of Chinese education*, New York, Teachers' College Press, Columbia University, 1969, pp. 27, 27–28, 34
5. Orleans, L. A. *Health policies and services in China, 1974. Prepared for the Subcommittee on Health of the Committee on Labor and Public Welfare, United States Senate*, Washington, D.C., United States Government Printing Office, 1974, p. 2
6. Ma Hai-teh. With Mao Tse-tung's thought as the compass for action in the control of venereal diseases in China. *China's Medicine*, No. 1: 52–68 (1966)
7. Horn, J. W. *Away with all pests... An English surgeon in People's China*, New York, Monthly Review Press, 1971, pp. 96, 126
8. A great victory of Mao Tse-tung's thought in the battle against schistosomiasis. *China's Medicine*, No. 10: 588–602 (1958)
9. Experience in health work and disease prevention in Heilungkiang Province in the past year. *China's Medicine*, No. 3: 148–153 (1968)
10. Sidel, V. W. & Sidel, R. *Serve the people: observations on medicine in the People's Republic of China*, Boston, Mass., Beacon, 1974, Appx. G, H
11. Sidel, R. *Families of Fengsheng: urban life in China*, Baltimore, Penguin, 1974
12. Han Suyin. Family planning in China. In: Piotrow, P. T., ed. *Population and family planning in the People's Republic of China*. New York, Victor-Bostrom Fund and Population Crisis Committee, 1971, pp. 16–21
13. Sidel, R. *Women and child care in China: a firsthand report*, Baltimore, Penguin, 1973
14. Wegman, M. E. Addendum: Some firsthand observations: June 15–July 6, 1973. In: Wegman, M. E. et al., ed. *Public health in the People's Republic of China*, New York, Josiah Macy Jr Foundation, 1973, p. 278
15. *Child health care in New China*, Peking, Chinese Medical Association, 1973 (republished in *American Journal of Chinese Medicine*, 2:149–158 (1974)).
16. Lamm, S. H. and Sidel, V. W. Public health in Shanghai: an analysis of preliminary data. In: Quinn, J. R., ed. *China medicine as we saw it*, Washington, D.C., Fogarty International Centre, 1974

THE NATIONAL HEALTH SYSTEM IN CUBA

ARNALDO F. TEJEIRO FERNANDEZ [a]

The original situation

The existence of a national health system in Cuba is a relatively recent phenomenon, a consequence of the changes that took place in the country after the Revolution in 1959. During the past two centuries Cuba has had hygienists and physicians who were remarkable specialists with outstanding achievements to their credit. At the national level, for example, Dr Thomas Romay introduced smallpox vaccination in Cuba just a few years after the experiments of Jenner; at the international level, the Cuban scientist Carlos Finlay made fundamental discoveries in connexion with the vector of yellow fever. These successes, however, did not go beyond personal triumphs and were but small achievements in limited spheres, not resulting in the intensive development of national activities in the health sector.

Finlay himself, the first leader of Cuban public health in the newborn Republic when the country had just been liberated from Spanish domination, did achieve in the first decade of this century some progress in the control of communicable diseases such as smallpox, plague, and yellow fever, and in particular the reduction of tetanus neonatorum, which was a scourge at that time.

This progress, however, did not continue. After that generation of physicians had disappeared, the country having been occupied on several occasions by foreign powers and national politics having become incredibly corrupt, the deterioration of Cuban public health continued until the 1950s. At this time it seemed that one feature characterized everything—a general incapacity to solve the majority of existing health problems. In the years before 1959 most of the population, especially those living in the rural areas, did not have ready access to health services of any kind. The state health services were inadequate and inefficiently organized and hardly covered the major cities; private pharmacists, traditional healers, and

---

[a] In collaboration with E. Liisberg, Division of Family Health, World Health Organization, Geneva, Switzerland.

"quacks" provided services for part of the population in the rural areas and in the small towns. Traditional birth attendants dealt with deliveries.

Apart from the deficient government services, other health institutions existed to cater for selected groups of industrial workers. Private hospital centres, in return for a monthly prepayment, gave services to the members of the so-called *mutualismos*. Numerous private clinics in the large and medium-sized cities, some of them converted residential houses, functioned as 8- or 10-bed "hospitals" under substandard conditions. Others were luxury clinics, generally well endowed with material resources, in the capital city of Havana.

There were also private institutions managed by charity groups and some hospital services run by various religious denominations. This completed the range of existing services, practically all of which were only of a curative nature. Prevention hardly found a place in this situation. Only people in extreme hardship used the government services. Indeed, when someone already beyond his first youth was not given to saving or providing for his own future or was unemployed or unmarried, it was frequently said that this unhappy person would end his days in a government hospital, as if that were the worst thing that could happen to anyone.

The private services were in general of better quality than the government ones, but they were expensive and a sizeable part of the population could not afford them. Besides, no effective control was exercised over them.

In the country as a whole there were in 1958 about 28 000 hospital beds, of which only 10 000 belonged to the government. Havana, with 22% of the population, accounted for 54.7% of the total beds. We could summarize all this by saying that the first and perhaps the most important deficiency was the absence of a national system of health care. But this was not the only problem. Between 200 and 300 physicians graduated from the medical school of Havana every year. Most of them decided to stay in the capital city to exercise their profession in the, very often substandard, private sector because the difference in living standards between the capital and the rest of the country was very great. Some settled in provincial capitals or in larger towns; invariably a large number emigrated every year to neighbouring countries, from where they usually did not return. This caused an imbalance in the distribution of physicians within the country; the city of Havana permanently had more than half of all the physicians in the country.

Between the year 1728, when the Havana Medical School was created, and the time of the Socialist Revolution (a period of more than 230 years) nobody thought of establishing, or at least nobody succeeded in establishing, even on a profit-making basis, an additional medical school in another province. Because they all worked in the large cities it seemed as if there was a surplus of physicians; only one in six doctors worked for the State, and even taking into account those working in private services there was quite a high level of unemployment among these professionals.

The conceptual basis of the approach adopted

The present Cuban experience in the field of health is based upon the result of the profound changes that have taken place in the whole social, political, and economic structure of the country since the Revolution in 1959. The essential health problems of the people and some of the ways of solving them were stated by the First Secretary of the Cuban Communist Party and Prime Minister of the Revolutionary Government, Commander Fidel Castro, in the document entitled "History will absolve me" in 1953.

From the beginning of this new era health and education have been accorded high priority by the Government. Together with agricultural and livestock development, with industrialization, and with improving the means of communication, health and education have been the pillars upon which the social and economic development of the country have stood during these historical fifteen years.

In Cuba, health is considered as one of the fundamental human rights and health services are free for everyone. Although there are still some differences between the various provinces, a permanent objective is to achieve an equal distribution of services as soon as possible. At the beginning this enterprise seemed gigantic in its proportions in contrast to the apparent simplicity of the basic socialist principles.

The first of these principles is that the health of the population is an unavoidable responsibility of the State. In order to fulfil this obligation the health services must be at the disposal of the whole population without any limitations. Taking into account the circumstances prevailing in Cuba at that particular time, the services had to be free since otherwise there was a risk that they might not be used. Therefore professional visits, complementary examinations, hospitalization, drugs for hospitalized patients, and special programmes and campaigns were all to be free. Other basic principles were those related to the preparation and participation of the people in health tasks and the integration of the services in a holistic preventive/curative programme.

The implementation of the above principles required careful planning, taking into account the specific characteristics of the country as well as other countries' experience. It was also indispensable to consolidate the statistical system to provide total coverage of continuous information, and a close surveillance was undertaken of the collection and quality of the primary data, to avoid the possibility of self-deceit.

15

Cuba has not been alone in the fulfilment of this objective. She has received the fraternal collaboration of other socialist countries, and particularly the Soviet Union. The World Health Organization has provided assistance both directly and through its Regional Office for the Americas. UNICEF has also collaborated in several ways to meet Cuba's needs. In addition, other countries have collaborated to a greater or lesser degree.

The action taken

From the outset it was considered necessary to integrate all the formerly separate components into a single organization able to give direction, set standards, and control all health activities—the Ministry of Public Health. As a consequence of the application of this principle all institutions in the medical field, including those formerly in the private sector, as well as the industrial and commercial undertakings concerned with drugs, were incorporated into this single health organization. This was a long process, completed only in 1970, when the *mutualismo* institution was incorporated and its services made available to the entire population.

The first institutions to be integrated into the Ministry of Public Health were those abandoned by their owners, who had left the country for various reasons. Most of the small private clinics run by groups of 3–4 doctors were voluntarily closed and reconverted into private homes because the services they provided were not up to the standards set by the Ministry; the physicians concerned were happy to accept Government posts with adequate salaries.

As from 1 August 1961, the Minister of Public Health became responsible, by law, for all public health services. The whole process was gradually carried out over a period of a few years because the Government had to create conditions for the continuous functioning of institutions after they had been taken over.

The private practice of medicine has also decreased. New graduates, in successive meetings from their early student days, have renounced the private practice of the profession. Salaries for physicians have been carefully established with due regard to the degree of specialization, and employment is guaranteed to every graduate in medicine (as in any other occupation). At present only about 350 doctors out of a total of 8 000 still have their private surgeries, and 200 of these also work half-time for the Government. The situation in the dental profession is similar.

At the same time, measures were adopted to achieve complete geographical and population coverage in the whole country. It was necessary to regionalize, centralizing policy and decentralizing implementation, with the purpose of making the organization more flexible and efficient. In each of the seven provinces the central organizational pattern is reproduced, excluding, of course, functions belonging properly to the national level, such as international relationships and the National Centre for Information on Medical Sciences. The next level is called the "health region", of which there are 43; these are divided into "areas", 332 purely executive divisions each covering some 30 000 people, each area being further subdivided into sectors (see Fig. 1). The area level was the most difficult one to establish.

FIG. 1. DIAGRAM SHOWING THE REGIONALIZATION OF HEALTH SERVICES IN CUBA

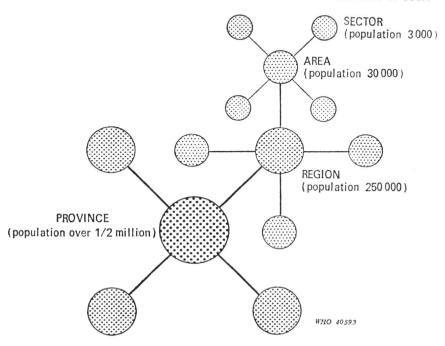

SECTOR
(population 3 000)

AREA
(population 30 000)

REGION
(population 250 000)

PROVINCE
(population over 1/2 million)

WHO 40593

An internationally famous incident—the missile crisis of October 1962—helped in this task since it necessitated, as a defence measure, the urgent sectorization of the country. Semi-autonomous units were created for a number of activities. The responsibility for comprehensive health services was assigned to a single unit. This structure, with some modification, was maintained afterwards and it corresponds to the present regional level. The regions were later divided into areas. In each area there is an integrated executive unit, a polyclinic in urban areas, and a hospital with 30–100 beds in rural areas, especially in mountainous areas.

Areas were selected for pilot studies on the maternal and child health programme, communicable diseases, environmental sanitation, food hygiene, occupational health, health education, and stomatology; the results of these studies were available within six months. A malaria eradication

17

programme has been in progress since 1960. Immunization schedules were established for the whole population, as well as gastroenteritis and tuberculosis programmes. Special attention was paid to aspects of maternal and infant mortality. These activities were extended to all parts of the country.

All this represents an immense effort. It is not easy to build and equip dozens of hospitals in the lowlands and in the mountains and dozens of polyclinics in the more populated areas, where the former facilities were either inadequate or all grouped together in a single area, as in the big cities. No less effort was required to prepare the necessary manpower. There was no point in building hospitals and polyclinics without, at the same time, preparing the staff to man them.

Before the Revolution, physicians had been trained exclusively to treat sick people and although they had humanitarian feelings they nevertheless looked upon medicine as a way of earning a living—and in some cases of amassing a fortune. Now, completely new and different horizons opened up before them in which health as a human right and a government obligation gave a new and wide social dimension to their work. Many did not appreciate the new concept and in the 1960s about 2500 physicians left the country to work abroad.

From 1959, however, other physicians began to volunteer to work for a time in the mountains, where no doctor had ever practised, except for some physicians during the Revolutionary War, Commander Ernesto Ché Guevara among them. They sowed the seed of what in the following years would become the rural medical social service and were replaced by the new graduates who had to give this service for a period of six months, later extended to two years.

As will be easily understood, a difficult situation existed in the beginning. The departure of physicians was not instantaneous but continued over a period of years. Those who stayed redoubled their efforts and the new leaders took immediate measures to train new physicians. The acute shortage of physicians resulting from the departures did not affect towns and rural areas in the same manner, because, as mentioned above, medical care was in any case very poor in the rural areas and non-existent in the mountains.

When rural hospitals were being built, the doctors settled where they could; farmers offered parts of their homes and everybody wanted the doctor in their house. Sometimes, part of a small grocery on some crossroad between the small farms was used as a rural health post for one, two or more years until the new installation was ready for use. When the, technical equipment imported from the USA broke down or became obsolete, the total blockade imposed on Cuba prevented the purchase of spare parts or new equipment. X-ray machines, anaesthetics apparatus, and electrocardiographs had to be thrown away because not a single screw could be obtained to repair them.

18

Valuable assistance from Socialist countries permitted the slow replacement of equipment.

But even these formidable difficulties could not daunt a people that had decided to change the course of its history.

All the rural hospitals and polyclinics for small communities could not be created in one, two, or even five years, nor could the health staff be trained overnight. Since many communities all over the country were requesting their own doctor and their own health establishment, it was necessary to explain to the people through mass organizations and mass media that everything was being implemented according to a plan giving equal attention to all. During these first five or six years, frequent meetings were also held with health staff at all levels from local to national level in order to review the situation in each place.

In 1962 a new medical school was created in Oriente, the easternmost province of the country, 1000 km from Havana. In 1965 a third medical school, not including a dental school, was established in Las Villas in the central province. In 1971 the new generation of graduates from these three schools was already able to balance more or less the deficit created by the emigration of doctors.

The situation as regards auxiliary and paramedical personnel was rather different. There were six training schools for nurses in the country, but personnel in laboratories, clinics, X-ray departments, and sanitation stations received only empirical in-service instruction. It was therefore necessary to create a whole new teaching structure for auxiliary personnel and middle-level technicians. The schools created throughout the country were distributed according to the requirements at the national, provincial, and regional levels. Between 1960 and 1973, 44 500 persons graduated from 26 nursing schools, hospital courses for nursing auxiliaries, and auxiliaries' and technicians' courses in clinical laboratory work, radiography, statistics, microbiology, stomatology, etc.

The production, distribution, and sale of pharmaceutical products in Cuba, as well as the maintenance of all facilities and equipment, is also the responsibility of the Ministry of Public Health, and the necessary personnel had to be trained by the Government.

The whole population was enrolled in the fight against diseases. A massive channelling of womenfolk into socially useful work has made a great contribution in this respect. In the first place, the free availability of all the mass media of the country, including radio, press, and television, facilitates an approach to the people. The reasons for each health activity are explained. Secondly, each member of every health team is prepared for a community approach as a health educator or orientation-giver. The new physician is also trained in contact with the community from the first year of his studies. At the local level, be it the rural hospital or polyclinic, people's health commissions are active. These commissions are presided over by the physician-director of the institution and each one of the mass organizations or community organizations is represented, such as the Committees for the Defence of the Revolution, the Federation of Cuban Women, and the labour unions. In the rural areas a member of the National Association of Small Farmers, who belongs to the private sector, is also a participant in the people's health commissions. The team is completed by a representative of the Communist Party. It meets regularly to consider a great diversity of problems, such as schoolchildren's vaccination and the hygiene of local milk production.

From the very first years following the Revolution, each of these grass-roots committees included a person responsible for health.

The Committees for the Defence of the Revolution started in 1960 in factories and in streets to fight against internal and external sabotage. Their coverage of the whole country and their enthusiasm made it possible very soon to give them other functions. Among the first were those related to public health; others were related to education and voluntary labour. Year after year the functions have been increasing.

In the field of public health, the first task, in conjunction with the health services, was the immunization of the whole population. Other important activities were the removal of animals from near houses and the elimination of rubbish, to avoid the proliferation of flies and other disease carriers.

The Committees for the Defence of the Revolution group together over three and a half million adults. Their primary level of organization corresponds to city blocks in the urban areas and to each large farm in the rural areas. The use of such an organization makes it possible to vaccinate one and a half million children with oral poliomyelitis vaccine in a few hours at almost no expense.

The tasks have been of increasing complexity. One example is voluntary blood donation to hospitals—and also to other countries in the case of disasters. To carry out these tasks, there is a structure similar to those of other mass organizations. Fifteen to thirty committees (in total there are more than 35 000 in the country) form a zone. Four to eight zones form a section, which in turn belongs to a region and a province in accordance with the administrative divisions of the country. At the top of the pyramid is the national direction.

Blood donation provides an example of the way in which the organization works. At the national level coordination is undertaken between the Committee and the Ministry of Public Health. A one-page document is prepared in simple language, printed in thousands of copies in provinces and regions, and sent to each committee, which then calls a meeting of its 20-30 or more member families in order to explain the matter. Generally, every family sends at least one representative. The meetings are held in various homes in rotation. In the case of emergency, infrequent in the last few years, the person responsible for health (one of the members of a family, elected by acclamation yearly) visits every house under his responsibility to inform everybody. The need for blood donation and its importance have been explained—how it helps save lives and how it is given free to those who need it. Each committee generally provides one donor every 6 months. There is no commerce in blood in the country.

In other cases matters taken up by the newpapers are discussed, the opinion of the committee is given in writing, and opinions are consolidated at each superior level up to the national level. This happens in the case of all social and labour laws, not only in the Committees for the Defence of the Revolution, but also in the labour unions, ensuring that the opinion of the masses influences the final form of the laws.

This kind of work—year after year—has created health consciousness among the population. The farmers and the women in the most remote areas of the country are enthusiastic about their present medical care and remember with sadness how—many years ago—they saw a son or a mother die without any medical attention at all; they all seem to have some sad story to tell about the old days.

Nowadays, when the public health staff carry out field surveys from house to house they explain the reasons for their visit in simple terms and are well received. Resistance or refusal is infrequent, even in surveys on fertility, when questions are asked on intimate problems of sexual life.

Older doctors who remember the past are astonished at what can be accomplished when people believe in their Government and are willing to participate in profound transformations.

Various similar health tasks undertaken by the Federation of Cuban Women may be mentioned. A pilot study of a broader plan of health activities drawn up by this Federation has recently been carried out. The results of this study, in conjunction with the experience acquired during the 10 years of the Federation's existence, were incorporated in the preparation of proposals now under study. The essence of these proposals is the training within the Federation, by means of 3-week courses, of enough health workers to ensure the provision of one or more workers, functioning within their own neighbourhood, for every 300 inhabitants.

The tasks of these workers include visiting the homes of women during pregnancy and the puerperium and follow-up visits for children discharged from hospital after suffering from diarrhoeal, acute respiratory, and other conditions. The workers ensure attendance for antenatal and child care at the health centres. They check that the hygiene, diet, and therapy prescribed on discharge are observed and that children receive the recommended immunizations. They also assess the mothers as regards hygiene in the home, feeding, and lactation and keep them informed of what the health service offers, thus ensuring better utilization of facilities.

These functions are undertaken in accordance with methods standardized throughout the country and in close cooperation with the local health centre and its district nursing staff. The health workers may be students, house-wives, retired women, or other kinds of workers devoting their spare time to these activities. The only requirement is a willingness to cooperate in the work.

This new form of community participation in health matters, promoted by the Federation but without interfering in the tasks of the various mass organs, stimulates the activities and training of the population in improving its own health and extends the total care offered by the health centre.

During the very first years of the new regime specialist task forces were organized. Each task force is made up of experts and university professors, who participate, in close collaboration with Ministry staff, in health planning in their own specialty. There are as many groups as there are specialties. Besides having planning responsibilities, some members of these groups also have directive functions at national or provincial level and in every case they have a role of direct supervision of yearly programmes, even down to the level of the executive unit.

In 1962 an epidemiological meeting established the minimum standards of diagnosis for communicable diseases occurring in the country, as well as of other epidemiological aspects for which it was necessary to unify criteria. In 1963 the obstetricians already working on clinical and thera-peutic matters drafted a manual of standards, or norms, which had an immediate success among doctors. These norms formed the basis of a development programme for the service units and led to partial standardiz-ation of the clinical work throughout the country, allowing for evaluation. Other norms were subsequently developed for surgery, internal medicine, and paediatrics.

The norms or standards are not a straightjacket, but, rather, guidelines as to what should correctly be done in each situation, considering the present state of science and the available resources. They do not determine or prejudge arguable questions or matters that are still doubtful, but concern only what can be considered as scientifically proven. In order to ensure their acceptance and their application it is necessary for practically all the specialists in the country to participate in the formulation of the norms. Details are distributed to provinces and regions by the national group months, or years, in advance. World literature and national experience are reviewed and finally hundreds of specialists from all over the country meet for 3–4 days to agree upon the norms. These are then printed in book form in thousands of copies and distributed to all concerned. From time to time they are reviewed and re-edited, so that modification is always possible. Medical students and other health trainees have discovered in these norms good learning material.

Strenuous efforts have been made to obtain the high-quality statistics required for immediate decision-making, health planning, and the evaluation process. Statisticians, as specialized staff, were hardly known fifteen years ago in Cuba. Since then 519 auxiliary statisticians, with one year of training after 8 years of basic education, have graduated, and 161 technicians, with 3 years of theory and practical preparation following completion of high school education, have also been trained. Over 20 physicians have chosen biostatistics as their specialty and are being prepared, in Cuba or elsewhere, to start major projects in research or in the services. Each unit, each region, and each province now has a statistical department.

Financing

In the years immediately following the Revolution the emergency was such that costs were considered a secondary matter. The revolutionary transformations had to be made at whatever price, since they were the very purpose of the Revolution. Health and education had always been considered by the leadership of the Revolutionary Government as absolute priorities and once they had been discussed and coordinated the total national development programmes were financed and budgeted on the basis of the decisions taken.

The health budget for 1968 (210 594 200 pesos) was almost ten times that for 1958 (22 670 000 pesos). This means that the government medical expenditure increased by 3.5 pesos *per capita* in 1958 to 27.3 pesos in 1968. Of course, because of the great difference between the circumstances in these two years the figures are not directly comparable. The combined budgets for health, education, and development of communications is a major part of the national budget, because the central leadership of the Revolution realizes that it is only on the very solid basis of those aspects that a more prosperous and happy future for the people can be built. All health services are paid for by the State. There are no other payments, taxes, or contributions from charitable institutions. The participation of the Red Cross, however, and of community or mass organizations, provides considerable voluntary support for the health organization.

In order to take into account the concept of cost efficiency, the financing of each activity is constantly being studied, not as a limitation to present development trends but rather as a planning tool that might permit achievement of the same result through a better utilization and distribution of resources, human as well as material and financial.

The progress made

The health services cover practically the entire population. The structure of the services is shown in Fig. 2. The utilization of these services also approaches 100%. The number of hospital beds grew from 28 500 in

1958 to 41 000 in 1973. The increase in beds in the most needy of all the provinces has been 100.5% in 15 years, compared with only 1.8% in Havana, the capital province. The planned 56 new rural hospitals have

FIG. 2. STRUCTURE OF THE REGIONALIZED HEALTH SERVICES IN CUBA

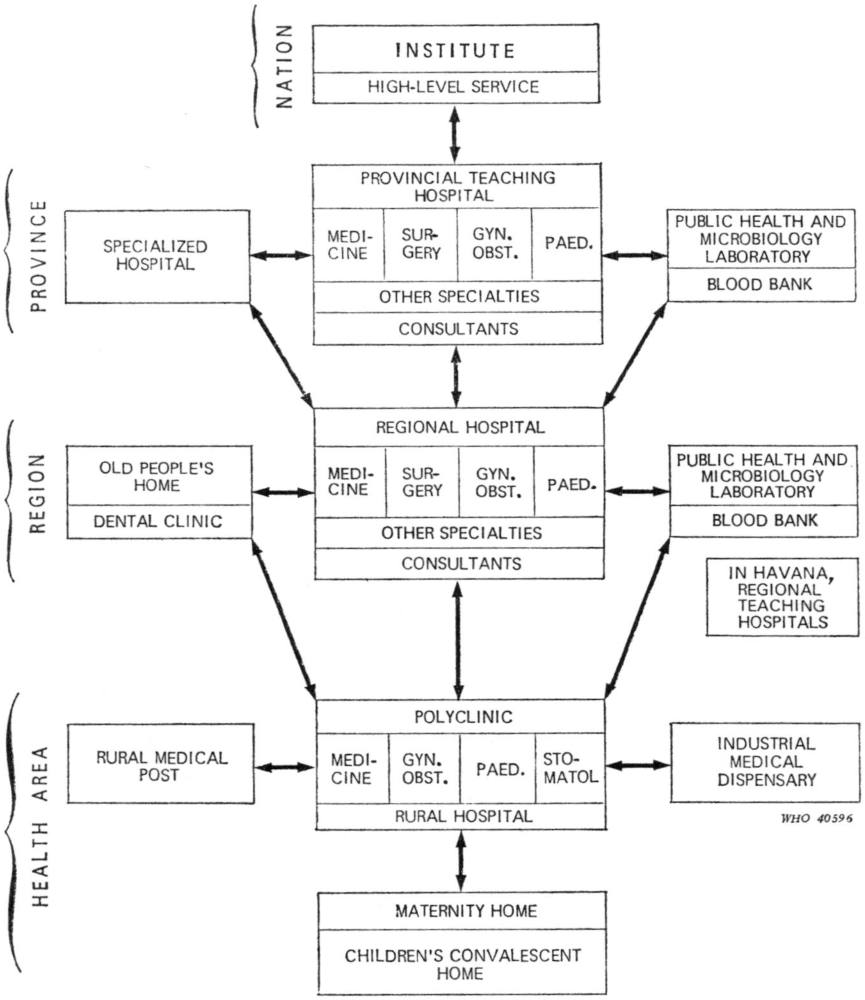

already been completed and each one staffed with 2–4 physicians, 1 stomatologist, 1 nurse, 8–10 nursing auxiliaries, laboratory technicians, X-ray technicians, an auxiliary or technician in pharmacy, a sanitation worker, and a statistician, as well as an administrator, an ambulance driver, and the general service workers. The number of doctors and nurses in the 322 area polyclinics is greater; the anticipated manpower is almost always available. The staffing will be completed as new students finish their studies.

In the capitals of the seven provinces there are general hospitals with 400–1000 beds; there are 6 in Havana, as well as maternity and children's hospitals. In each one of the 43 regions there is a general hospital with 150–450 beds. Just over half of the regions have specialized maternity and children's hospitals. In the rest of the regions obstetric and paediatric services are provided in the general hospitals.

Except for neurology, which is mostly available at provincial level, and some other specialties requiring a low doctor/population ratio, all the specialties function at the level of the region. This facilitates the reference of cases from the base. Great use is made of this referral system; the cases can be sent to a province or referred directly to a region, depending on their complexity and the need for care. At the highest scientific echelon there are, in Havana, 10 specialized institutes, which are available for patients requiring this high level of care, wherever they may live in the country.

A policy that has given good results is that every institution complying with the established standard is recognized as a teaching institution for the final years of medical studies and for the internship period, or for the period of residence in a specialty (this period lasts for 2–4 years and is undertaken after the graduate has completed his rural service). All provincial hospitals and some regional hospitals now offer such teaching. Institutions that do not meet the standard (medical qualification, type of facilities or resources) aspire to do so and are working to that end.

The regional and provincial specialists regularly offer, in the polyclinics, outpatient consultations in their specialities. Doctors in rural hospitals and polyclinics are in constant contact with units at higher level. Further training and improvement is available to all doctors in the country and they all receive regular technical information through the National Centre for Information on Medical Sciences, which maintains an exchange of publications with a great number of countries in the world. There is an urgent need to computerize the cumbersome work of providing information and bibliographies and to simplify the preparation of summaries.

The medical profession has been transformed and the curative doctor of former times has been replaced by a professional with a wide comprehensive concept of medicine, to whom the whole range of aspects—from primary prevention or environmental change through medical care to rehabilitation—are of equal concern. Close contact with the community is being achieved, although there is still room for improvement in this respect.

No method has yet been found to prepare a physician, within the present concept of such a professional, in less than six years after the completion of pre-university studies.

The yearly number of visits to the physician per inhabitant has increased from 1.9 in 1963 to 3.9 in 1973 and stomatological visits from 0.1 in 1963 to 0.6 in 1973.

In 1973 there were, on average, 8.5 antenatal visits per pregnant woman, and child health supervision visits, which began only in 1967, are now at the level of 4.5 per infant per year. These services, it should be emphasized, are equally available in the central section of the city of Havana and in the mountains of the eastern province.

Especially outstanding are the achievements in the institutional assistance of deliveries—slightly more than 96% of all births in the country in 1973. We believe that this has had a great impact on the reduction of maternal mortality, which in 10 years has decreased from 12 to 5.5 per 10 000 deliveries. It must also have had an influence in the reduction of infant mortality—28.7 per 1 000 live births in 1972 and less than 28 in 1973.

Mortality from infectious diseases has been markedly reduced in the revolutionary period. The gastroenteritis mortality rate fell from 58.1 per 100 000 persons in 1962 to 9.7 in 1973. The mortality rate for tuberculosis was 19.6 per 100 000 in 1962 and 4.1 in 1973. The mortality rate for measles, which was 1 per 100 000 population in the first years of the decade, is now 0.2 per 100 000. Poliomyelitis has been practically eradicated; its incidence, which was 200–400 cases per year in the early 1960s, has fallen to only 3 cases in the last 9 years—all children who for some reason had not been vaccinated. The eradication of malaria was completed in June 1967. The incidence of diphtheria averages only 2–3 cases a year, and no case has appeared since 1971. The control programmes for leprosy and tuberculosis are now close to detecting and giving medical care for all cases estimated to exist in the country. The pattern of other diseases is changing more slowly but the trend is always towards a reduction, which serves as a stimulus to continue the work.

It would not be honest to present these important fundamental aspects of the development and the progress of the health system in Cuba as an isolated phenomenon unrelated to their social context. This would give a false picture since decisive factors have influenced all the aspects so far covered.

Education, for example, has been given the same priority as health, and in 1959 the eradication of illiteracy was begun. Every child of school age in the country goes to school. The working people have also been massively enrolled in the classrooms in each factory and in every industry, even during working hours.

Education is free, with all the necessary books, from the preschool age up to and including the university, and an average of 250 000 yearly scholarships are awarded to intern students. This situation greatly facilitates health activities. The law strictly forbids the employment of school-age children; their first obligation is to study.

The complete radio, television, and press coverage of the country, the easy access of the health sectors to this communication system, and the existence of a literate population who can understand the message are all of considerable value in facilitating health activities.

Complete employment (even shortage of manpower), the employment of women in social work on equal conditions with men, the construction throughout the country of small rural villages of up to 500 houses with all necessary services (water supply, schools, medical services, sewerage, and electric light) to replace the poor isolated village houses—all this means as much for the health situation, we believe, as the most important measures in the health field proper. The elimination of miserable quarters at the periphery of large cities—one of the first activities of the Revolution—has resulted in the almost complete disappearance of the so-called peripheral zone of pathological urbanism, this terrible urban agglomeration with some rural characteristics. The increase in the paved road network of the country, from about 4500 kilometres in 1958 to 22 300 kilometres now, has greatly contributed to the health of the population; we say without shame that some of the first mountain hospitals built in places that could be reached only by mule were already obsolete 6, 8, or 10 years later when roads were built making populated centres with more resources accessible from such places by means of a bus ride of about half an hour. Some of these mountain hospitals have been replaced by simple medical posts.

Perhaps even more decisive for health is the fair distribution of food to the whole population. It is frequently asked what is the contribution to the decrease in infant mortality of giving one litre of milk per day to each Cuban child up to seven years of age. Milk, by the way, is also given to elderly people. Equally, what has been the contribution of protein consumption, which, in terms of fish only, has increased from 21 500 metric tons in 1958 to 139 890 metric tons in 1972?

The present position

Many of the fundamental elements of the national health system have now been established, but there is still room for improvement. We speak with enthusiasm of our progress and our statistics, but with the attitude not of people who have achieved their goals but of people who pause to evaluate, to think, to harvest experience, and to summon new energy in order to forge ahead.

Public health planning is now being undertaken over a longer term and always in coordination with the socioeconomic planning of the country. A plan covering the period up to the year 1980 has already been prepared. The present mortality and morbidity profile of Cuba deserves careful consideration, since communicable diseases have already become a very small problem whereas cardiovascular diseases are now the first cause of death and account for one quarter of the total mortality. Cancer and cerebrovascular accidents follow. Although life expectancy at birth in our country is around 70 years, the analysis of the age distribution of the above-mentioned causes of death shows that there is already an important incidence of this pathology at an early age.

Since 1970 research on population morbidity has been carried out; arterial hypertension, bronchial asthma, and diabetes mellitus will be the object of special projects. The control of accidents, particularly traffic accidents, also requires coordination and joint activities between health and other bodies.

In the immediate future some population groups, especially school-children, will receive particular attention with regard to sensory capacity or acuity, orthopaedic problems, psychological problems, and retardation of learning. Another priority group is the workers; the study of national standards of acceptability for noise, vibration, toxic gases, and other hazards is necessary in order to deal with the problems created by industrialization.

We have placed great hopes in three large research projects that started two or three years ago. The first is concerned with the growth and development of a carefully designed, randomized sample of 56 000 persons under 20 years of age. Fifteen anthropometric measurements, including weight and height, will allow us to estimate Cuban patterns and standards of growth. The execution phase of this investigation, requiring two years of work all over the country, has already been completed. We hope one day to cease measuring sickness and to measure only health.

The second research study relates to all births occurring in one week in Cuba, all low-weight births in one month, and all perinatal deaths over a 3-month period. This investigation includes the post-mortem study of the perinatal deaths. As has happened in other countries, now that infant mortality has fallen below 30—35, half of the total infant mortality is occurring during the first week of life; studies of perinatal problems are therefore essential. The data collection for this research is already accomplished.

The third investigation concerns indicators of human and physical resources relating to the total morbidity of a population. It is now in the field phase.

Some work is also being done in connexion with the subject of consumer satisfaction, or community satisfaction, with the services provided, and the criteria used by the community to establish their needs are being explored.

Home visits by physicians in cases of emergency or sudden illness are now being increased, particularly for children and elderly people. Communities do not readily accept having to bring the sick members of these two age groups, for example, a fever case, to the health facility. They prefer at least the first medical consultation to take place in the home. The pilot stage of this project has already been completed and it is now being extended to the services in several provincial capitals.

In the first months of 1974 the Ministry asked the Pan American Health Organization for consultants to visit and review our statistical system, particularly in relation to childhood and maternity. We wished to learn about other people's experiences and criteria. An expert sent in March 1974 visited hospitals and studied registers and files; she interviewed doctors and her report resulted in a request from the Director of the Pan-American Health Organization to the Director of the Statistical Office of the United Nations to the effect that from now onwards any indication of incompleteness or low quality in the Cuban health statistics as published in the demographic year book be discontinued since health statistics in Cuba are now complete and reliable.

Finally we may repeat that the Revolutionary Government continues to give the highest priority to the health of the people.

FURTHER READING

Cuba, Ministerio de Salud Pública. *Informe de la República de Cuba a la III Reunión Especial de Ministros de Salud de las Américas*, Havana, 1972

Cuba, Ministerio de Salud Pública. *Organización de los servicios de salud materno-infantiles y dinámica de población*, Havana, 1973

Cuba, Ministerio de Salud Pública, Organización de los Servicios y Nivel de Salud. *Informe a la XXVI Reunión Anual de la Sociedad Mexicana de Salud Pública*, Havana, 1972

Rojas Ochoa, F. *La Regionalización de los servicios de salud*, Havana, 1960

Navarro, V. Health service in Cuba: an initial appraisal. *New Engl. J. Med.*, **287**: 954 (1972)

The Lancet and Nuffield Provincial Hospital Trust. *Health Service Prospects. An International Survey*, London, 1973

Cuba, Ministerio de Salud Pública. *Anuario Estadístico, 1973* (in press).

Pan American Health Organization. Antecedentes del Plan Quadrienal, Washington, 1974

Puffer, R. R. *Informe acerca de la calidad y cobertura de las estadísticas vitales y sobre investigaciones de mortalidad perinatal e infantil en Cuba*, Pan American Health Organization, Washington, D. C., 1974

THE CHIMALTENANGO DEVELOPMENT PROJECT IN GUATEMALA

CARROLL BEHRHORST [a]

For 12 years we have lived and worked with the Cakchiquel Indians of Guatemala, a proud, dignified, life-loving but impoverished people whose cultural heritage stems from the great Mayan civilization, which lavished its artistic and architectural riches through Central America and the Yucatan peninsula of Mexico in the centuries before the Spanish conquest 450 years ago.

We have gone to school with the Cakchiquels, letting them teach us (myself—a North American doctor trained in the complex technology of modern medicine—and my companions) the simplicities of what the Cakchiquels believe they need to live and prosper in the highlands of Guatemala, where 3 000 000 agrarian Indians eke out a bare existence beneath the slumbering volcanoes that dominate this land of majestic beauty and sordid poverty.

We have learned more from our Indian friends than they have learned from us and we have come to believe that much of what we have absorbed here has wide application to the rural poor throughout the world. Certainly, what we saw and heard on a survey of mission hospitals in Africa and Asia in 1972 (for the United Presbyterian Church in the USA) confirmed our suspicion that the problems and indicated solutions in Guatemala were duplicated widely elsewhere. Despite differences of culture, language, and race the rural poor of all continents share a common bond forged of poverty, exploitation, disease, malnutrition, and land hunger. As a result of our "student days" with the Cakchiquels and our recent travels among peoples facing a similar battery of problems, we have reached a number of conclusions concerning the great public health question of the day—how to break the back of disease among the almost 2 000 million rural poor in the less developed regions of the world.

The old answer was a simple one: "We will eradicate disease by curing the sick". It was also a deceptive answer that brought balm to the spirits

---

[a] In collaboration with E. P. Mach, Division of Strengthening of Health Services, World Health Organization, Geneva, Switzerland.

of millions of donors in the industrialized countries while wasting hundreds of millions of dollars and untold mental energy. No sooner was the patient cured than he returned to a slough of poverty that once again felled him within months, often within days, of his treatment. Curing the ailing from clinics and hospitals located in jungles, savannas, and mountains was something like trying to empty the Atlantic Ocean with a teaspoon. It made the toiler feel active and useful and caused everyone to exclaim: "My, what a beautiful teaspoon!"

Today our answer is at once more tentative and far more complex. Before health can supplant disease among the 2 000 million rural poor of the world, we believe that the following problems must be tackled aggressively. Our listing of priorities generally reflects the opinions and feelings of the people we serve:

1. Social and economic injustice
2. Land tenure
3. Agricultural production and marketing
4. Population control
5. Malnutrition
6. Health training
7. Curative medicine.

You will note that we list curative medicine as our last priority. Twelve years ago, when we arrived in Guatemala from a medical practice in Kansas, USA, we would have listed curing first. We learned the hard way—by personal experience. Our list may look formidable to you, so formidable that a beginning by a single individual or group would seem to be doomed from the start. Yet, impossible as the task may seem, we are convinced that a fruitful beginning can be made by individuals outside the health bureaucracies of the world. We are also convinced that with careful nurturing and persistence an impact for wider change can be made from the most humble and inexpensive start. We think we have proved it in Guatemala—although we have a long, long way to go yet. Let us describe the origin and evolution of our experiment in the Indian highlands.

These highlands of Guatemala are like many areas of the non-socialist Third World as seen through the lens of economic and public health statistics. They are predominantly agricultural and poor in resources, and the wealth that does exist is concentrated in the hands of an elite class. The gross national product is increasing, largely through farm exports, but the great mass of the people do not share in these benefits. The condition of the Cakchiquels, oppressed and exploited by the Spanish conquistadores and by more than 20 generations of their descendants, is reflected in the state of public health. The infant mortality rate is one of the highest in the world. Respiratory infections, malnutrition, and intestinal disorders are primary causes of death and many of the other diseases, such as measles, tuberculosis, whooping cough, and influenza, no longer considered threats in the industrialized countries, still stalk the ridges and remote valleys of the Guatemalan highlands. This is one of the few areas in Latin America where the pre-Columbian population (called "Indian") is predominant. This indigenous people, descendants of the ancient Maya, make up more than three-fourths of the inhabitants of the highlands. They have held tenaciously to their culture and with a high degree of success. This demands that work with them be done on their own terms, for they have little appetite to copy modern cultures.

How the project began

When we first came to Chimaltenango, the hub of the Indian highlands, in 1962, we did little but walk around town, get acquainted with the people, and play with the children. Gradually we were invited into their homes to have coffee with them or sit down to a meal of tortilla and beans. This went on for 3 months until we were well known and accepted in the town and until we felt confident that we could fulfil a need. Then we rented a building for US$25 a month and opened a clinic. The first day 125 patients came, and we have never had less than that number since (the average is now 200 a day). We were in the business of curing.

It did not take us long to realize that we were trying to empty, if not the Atlantic Ocean, at least a good-sized lake, with a medical teaspoon. We began to see the same patients returning after a few months with the same ailments and we began to wonder what we should do about it. While this is not the place to analyse our personal transformation, the basic change in our thinking and attitudes can be symbolized by what happened to Jorge.

We met Jorge about a year after coming to Chimaltenango. He was a handsome 5-year-old Indian boy, but he was suffering that day he came to the clinic with his mother. He had puffy eyes, swollen feet, pigmentation blemishes on his arms and legs, and stains the colour of port wine. Questioning Jorge and his mother, we found that he lived in the village of San Jacinto in the rugged mountain country near Chimaltenango. Since he was not the first child from San Jacinto to come in with this problem, we decided to go to the town and have a look at conditions there.

Several days later, with two nurses from the clinic, we drove to San Jacinto by jeep. Although the village is only 8 km from Chimaltenango, the journey was a long one. There was no road then and our jeep often became mired in mud holes. At last we left the vehicle and walked the rest of the way. The trouble in San Jacinto was not hard to diagnose. Almost every child we saw was malnourished and diarrhoea was common in both adults and children. A great deal of coughing could be heard. As we visited the thatch-roofed huts, we learned that the common diet

32

had very little protein. The village existed almost exclusively on tortillas and vegetables.

Why? The people had no land to farm, only miserable little plots in areas where the soil was poor. San Jacinto was almost completely surrounded by large plantations operated for the benefit of absentee owners. The poor of the village, seeking an opportunity to earn a bare living, customarily packed up once a year and went to work on the big coffee *fincas* on the Pacific Coast of Guatemala. Going from the cool highlands to the hot lowlands, they fell victim to a variety of tropical ailments and often many returned to their village with tuberculosis. In fact, when the two Indian nurses from our clinic made a house-to-house survey a few weeks after our visit, they found that of 450 people, 105 had active tuberculosis.

We realized that no matter how many times we treated Jorge and other youngsters from San Jacinto they would never be healthy until drastic changes were made in the village. We began in a small, tentative way. A Peace Corps volunteer attached to the clinic, Wayne Haage, made weekly visits to San Jacinto, gained the confidence of the men, and began to teach better farming methods to a group who tilled their small plots for survival. Later, our first chicken project was started in the village. We lent money from our initial operating funds to 25 families to raise chickens and produce eggs. Soon the people began to eat more protein—"an egg a day" became the slogan with some families. The loan was repaid in full, the borrowers giving us a portion of the egg production in lieu of cash.

Gradually our programme expanded in San Jacinto. One of our Cakchiquel health "promoters", trained by us in Chimaltenango, opened his own little clinic in the village and began treating the common ailments on a fee-for-service basis. At the villagers' request, our Indian extension workers from the Chimaltenango programme taught nutrition, health care, and farming methods. Ten families banded together and bought some land from one big absentee owner, using a small fund borrowed from us and paying us back conscientiously as crops began to bring a dribble of cash to the town. Now San Jacinto plans a major land-buying programme, to be carried out when we have accumulated the necessary land-loan revolving fund, which has as its source grants from various international foundations. The women of the village have organized a weaving club that brought in $3513 in the year 1973, a remarkable income when contrasted with the pitiful handful of coins that people earned a decade ago.

Today San Jacinto is a reasonably healthy, economically viable community. Malnutrition has all but disappeared and the dreaded tuberculosis has been eliminated. You can walk through the village today without hearing a single cough. Jorge himself is a robust teenager doing a man's work. While San Jacinto is still poor, it has a new vibrancy compounded of protein, cash, and hope. And that hope is no mirage. We are convinced that when the new revolving fund becomes available, more men of San Jacinto will become proud land-owners and that the little mountain town, once a scrap-heap of disease and apathy, will become a prosperous agricultural community. A Cakchiquel family can flourish on a few acres of its own land.

True, San Jacinto is not the world, but a million San Jacintos might transform the world. As our own programme has evolved over the years, we can see dozens of San Jacintos scattered through the Guatemalan highlands and we feel we are on the right track. In brief, what started as curing the sick has broadened into a general community development programme geared to the services that the people want and need and focused always on that ultimate goal—acquisition of farm land by the Indians. But despite the change in emphasis we have never neglected curative medicine. Indeed, without curing, our expanded programme would have been most difficult, probably even impossible, to achieve.

Our experience has hammered home an important truth on the tactics of developing similar programmes in impoverished areas. The man who does not plan ways of doing himself out of a job is not doing the job. Institutionalized charity from outside accomplishes little but the cosseting of the egos of the helpers. If the programme does not take root in native soil and native hands, it will wither the moment the foreign helper ceases his aid. The Cakchiquels receive no charity from us. They borrow at reasonable interest rates from us, they pay for the services they want, and they increasingly select the people they want to deliver those services. All of our health promoters are Indians, as are most of our nurses and extension workers. We shall consider our job completed the day a trained Cakchiquel doctor takes over our medical and administrative chores at the Chimaltenango clinic, hospital, and extension service.

Although the Indians in the Guatemalan highlands generally had accepted modern medicine because of the wide availability of drugs in pharmacies, they were nevertheless somewhat reluctant to accept our newly introduced service because of the cultural barrier. Gradually, however, we were able to identify with them and our services were readily accepted.

It was not difficult at this point for us to offer treatment on terms the local person could afford. Our work was being subsidized by the Lutheran Church and we had access to a good deal of free and discount medicines. But, obviously, if this arrangement were to continue indefinitely, the local people would continue to be dependent on outside aid that was not entirely reliable. Also it became apparent that other ways to cut costs and adjust conventional medical approaches were needed if more people were to be reached.

The hospital

Some illnesses needing prolonged treatment are best attended while the patient is in hospital, particularly if he lives at a great distance and is not able to travel back and forth daily. Conventional hospitals, however, are a very expensive proposition. Poor rural areas cannot afford the hotel services and elaborate facilities of modern hospitals. In fact, impressive buildings with sophisticated rules of procedure are almost certain to alienate the local people.

In Chimaltenango we decided to build a very modest hospital where the patient could stay with his or her family, who would be responsible for preparing food and providing basic patient care. This arrangement turned out to be not only far less expensive but also far more humane. If you visit our hospital today, you will find scores of patients attended by members of their own families; this eliminates the need for the complex hotel services that make the sophisticated hospital so costly to the patient.

Costs to the patient for all our hospital services, including medicine, work out at the equivalent of $0.75 per day. This payment does not quite cover all expenses, but that is because our hospital must function as a public hospital since it is the only hospital in the Department of Chimaltenango, which has more than 200 000 inhabitants. We must accept any and all patients (we would anyway) regardless of their ability to pay even the most modest charge. Also, we offer such ancillary services as ambulance and transport and this cuts into our budget.

Health promoters

We had to challenge some of the sacred institutions of modern medicine in order to meet the needs of the people on their own terms. Once we had reformulated the concept of "hospital", we went on to challenge "the doctor" himself. This is much more delicate ground. In most developed countries, people still believe that only a medical doctor with a degree acquired after long academic training is competent to cure even minor ailments. This is simply not true. Even in the industrialized countries the vast majority of patients are in no real need of a sophisticated doctor. The developed countries can ill afford to perpetuate the myth of the indispensable doctor—poor areas, such as rural Guatemala, plainly cannot afford the myth at all.

After the first couple of years of seeing 125–150 patients a day we began to realize that a bright Cakchiquel, given a certain amount of inexpensive training, could treat the most common afflictions just as well as a university-trained doctor. Not only would the investment in the education of this "health promoter" be far more modest in both time and finances, but the fact that the local health promoter could respond to the customs of his own people would be invaluable in terms of public health, the acceptability of modern medicine, and the development of other needed community services.

It should be emphasized that the concept of using community health promoters came about not only because of a vacuum of medical help and lack of medical professionals but also because it was genuinely felt that the work of a local community-rooted and community-oriented worker would be more readily accepted, and, in fact, the total task did not demand the very costly services of a technically trained physician.

The doctor/population ratio in rural Guatemala is variously stated, but the statistics need not be quoted since in most communities a professional medical service simply does not exist. Now the Government has an energetic programme of introducing medical students to rural areas. This may be a step in the right direction but its contribution towards meeting the total medical need is minimal, and in view of the current rapid population growth an even more vigorous programme would still fail to keep up with the expanding need.

So, in order to help meet the urgent needs in many medically neglected communities, we began to train responsible Indians from those communities how to recognize and alleviate common medical problems. This programme now comprises more than 70 health promoters from 50 communities, not including some individuals we have trained in intensive courses. The common problems here are quite simple, diarrhoea and pneumonia accounting for more than 75% of the patient visits to our clinic and hospital. Our trainees, or "promoters" as we call them, come from most areas of the Department of Chimaltenango, Solola, Sacatepequez, and Quiche. Their formal education ended, on the average, after the third grade of elementary school, but they are for the most part bright, eager to learn, and quite skilful at treating ailments within their competence. One day we took an American specialist in tropical medicine on a tour of some of the health promoters at work. He was sceptical that men with so little formal education could dispense adequate medical care, but as the day wore on and he found the promoters dealing knowledgeably with one ailment after another, his scepticism wilted. Finally, he thought he had caught one of the promoters giving incorrect treatment. "You have the right disease, but the wrong remedy", he said to the promoter. "The specific indicated here is penicillin." The Indian promoter shook his head. "Ah", he replied, "but this patient is allergic to penicillin."

We have found that it is of vital importance to select the trainees with care. At first we generally accepted those who were recommended to us by a local priest or a Peace Corps volunteer. We have since learned better. Our approach now is to encourage each community to set up a

36

community betterment committee, which includes a health committee. Then the community health committee selects the person whom we are to train. This works well and avoids some of the pitfalls characteristic of the medical monopoly in the developed countries. The man we train represents his community and the community is responsible for him and can discipline him, retain him, or recommend his dismissal. We had to withdraw one health promoter because his local health committee was unhappy with the way he was offering his services.

The local committee has a list of the prices of the medicines. Each promoter is expected to charge according to this price list. In addition, he can charge a fee of 25 cents for his call or for his services. Since the community is involved in setting the charges, it is less likely that a monopoly can develop such as that in the USA and other countries where the physician can generally charge whatever he likes. Since we wanted to avoid such a monopoly, we insisted that a community requiring a community health leader must first form a committee to be responsible for the promoter, both during his training and later.

Most promoters come once a week for either Tuesday or Friday sessions and spend the entire day with us. The day begins with hospital rounds to check patients with a doctor or the supervisor. The student sees the patient and his problem and learns how that problem could be handled in his home village and how it could be prevented in the future. We usually do not speak of diseases as such, but rather talk of the patient's symptoms, since symptoms have meaning while diseases do not.

We should like to emphasize our belief that any programme for training lay medical workers that does not include facilities for patient demonstration cannot be effective. Seeing a patient with an ailment is of more value than 6 hours of lectures. Films, books, pamphlets, and seminars all have their place, along with classroom lectures, but they are adjuncts to a living demonstration, not substitutes for it.

We are frequently asked how the local medical profession and the Government look upon our programme, since it obviously contradicts the idea cherished by the profession that only a physician can treat a patient. The answer is that they all tolerate the programme because of the sparsity of professional help in the deprived communities, or, as a visitor who is very interested in training lay medical workers recently told us: "The answer is simple. It works." Just now we are beginning to coordinate our entire medical programme within the structure of the local health department so that there will be no overlapping of services and we can present a united front. Included in the plan is a proposal to use our promoters as agents of various health and preventive programmes sponsored by the Department of Public Health. We have long been aiming towards this integration because we earnestly believe that any programme developed and evolved by a foreigner is of no permanent value unless it is eventually accepted, supported, and understood by the local government or other local agencies. We should never create anything that cannot be locally self-sustaining.

Our programme of health promoter training is a continuous one. Promoters are usually trained in groups, attending sessions once weekly for a year. A promoter may enter at any time. Nearly all of them, even those who began their training more than 8 years ago, still come every week to learn new techniques and treatments. A promoter must attend sessions for a minimum of a year before he is allowed to dispense medicines and give injections. We give at least monthly examinations in which each promoter must describe what he sees in a patient, what is to be done for the ailment, and what might be done in the patient's home to prevent a recurrence of the problem. Generally the promoters do quite well. On the last examination, given just before this was written, all gave better than acceptable answers, the majority being excellent. The promoters are visited regularly on the job by a supervisor, who consults and advises. The supervisor is one of the older promoters, an Indian who is in complete charge of the programme. He consults the doctor, or another professional, only when, in his opinion, the problem warrants it.

The Indian supervisor, Carlos Xoquic, is in complete charge of the continued training, supervision, and management of the community health promoter programme. What initially may have been a "one-man show", conceived and nurtured by an expatriate, is now completely in the hands of the local people, supervised by Carlos in his communal-type relationship with the other promoters. Promoters are encouraged to keep records on all patients and these records are checked by the field supervisor.

It should be noted that prior to the development of this health promoter programme in the Chimaltenango area there was not a complete vacuum of medical services. Modern medicine was empirically dispensed by a pharmacist, along with that of the *curanderos* (Indian curers), who delivered a mixture of traditional and modern therapy.

As noted earlier, modern medicines were generally available in pharmacies and, as in many places in the world, are still valuable for common ailments. *Curanderos* were generally few in number in our section of the Guatemalan highlands because of this acceptance of modern medicine. Two of the *curanderos* elected to upgrade their service in a sense and become promoters in our programme. One other local *curandero* who is well accepted by his community openly collaborates with us, referring unusual problems to our clinic, and we in turn send patients to him who need further follow-up and injections.

Since the promoters generally work with poverty-stricken people who often cannot at the moment afford to pay cash, a system of credit that is both effective and reliable has been developed by the promoters. The success of this system is the result of the culture of the highland Indian, where responsibility, respect, and honesty are all part of local tradition.

Although the health promoters were trained over a period of a year (coming one day per week) and were not allowed to undertake medical work during that time, they did engage in other community service work; they are trained in total community service and they were actively involved in work of this kind during their medical training period.

All medicine in the health promoter programme is bought locally in Guatemala City from drug manufacturers. The buying and selling of medicines is strictly business. Our clinic places the orders for the medicines, since we can buy at reduced hospital prices. All supplies are then passed on to the promoters' medicine cooperative at our price plus a 10% handling fee. The promoters have a three-man committee to regulate the buying and selling, one of the three being responsible for the mechanics of the sales. The medicine cooperative then sells directly to the promoters at the cooperative's purchase price, plus 5% for its expenses. Thus, medicine is available at reduced prices, much below those quoted in the pharmacies. This plan might not work in some countries where medicines are not available locally at reasonable prices.

Our promoters can buy only those medicines that we believe they can dispense with minimum risk to the patient. Any drug with potentially serious side effects cannot be bought or used. Adrenal corticosteroids and digitalis preparations, for instance, may not be included in the promoter's medicine chest.

We teach the promoter not only what he can do but also what he must not do. For example, an elderly man with swollen feet and shortness of breath probably has heart failure and the promoter must see that the man receives professional help, even if it means carrying him out of a village in a chair tied to a porter's back. The promoters are trained to identify and treat the majority of diseases in their villages. However, they all know the limits of their capacity and they refer difficult cases to the clinic in Chimaltenango or to another nearby health centre. One study of the effectiveness of our promoters showed a low percentage of error in treatment, about 9%. The study was made by the University of Kentucky's department of community medicine some 7 years ago. We are now planning a more elaborate survey to determine the exact quality of work of each promoter.

One point concerning the delivery of "care" to a patient is not generally understood, particularly by professionals. Since medical service generally is provided for those in need, it is thought that the patient should accept it gratefully, even if the service is not on his terms but on those of the provider. But medicine should be practised for the benefit of the patient, in a manner understood and acceptable to him, and with the patient participating in the decision-making on what is to happen to his health and his life. "Care" should be so dedicated and so delivered that the patient can help decide his own medical destiny. This, of course, has not been the case in most medical delivery systems.

Recently a medical man, after visiting one of our health promoters, asked why the promoter did not send his Indian patients to the local health centre since, said the doctor, the goal of any medical programme should be to bring professional care to the people. The fact that this health centre was staffed by non-Indians did not seem relevant to him. We replied that the promoters do collaborate with health centres where they exist, but it is for the patient himself to decide where he wants to be treated.

The same doctor, after spending a week training himself in the total programme and visiting first-hand the work of various promoters, came to understand why patients prefer treatment by the promoters to attending the health centre, and agreed with us that we should accept the patient's decision as to which type of treatment he should receive. In addition, he did not think it necessary to send the patients to the referral centre, since they were well cared for by the promoter.

In the highlands of Guatemala, large numbers of Indians prefer to be treated by their own kind, regardless of the degree of skilled training, rather than be attended by a non-Indian medical professional. This being the case, we honour the patient's wish to be served by whomever he wants and we, therefore, train the type of person the patient trusts and accepts. If this stings the pride and conceit of members of the doctors' guild, so be it. The monopoly of doctors has for centuries dictated to the patient what service he will receive. The fact that this system is traditional in the profession in no way makes it just, serviceable, or humane. Medicine needs a new watershed, a new tradition whereby technicians and professionals, together with the community, consider the people's needs and where they wish to go when they are sick. It is a tragic error to assume that the whole wide world is content to be treated (or mistreated) by highly schooled technocrats rather than by an unsophisticated person.

The following is an example of the local Indian people's preference for care from those of their own culture. In a large nearby Indian town, three types of medical service are available—a health centre staffed by non-Indian nurses and medical students, a local *curandero*, and two community health promoters. If local people are asked where they prefer to go when they are sick, the great majority say they prefer to be attended by either the *curandero* or the health promoters. In fact, a past mayor of the town said that he believed only about 5% of the population prefer to go to the professionally staffed health centre, the remaining 95% preferring the non-professionals.

The reason why non-professionals are preferred to professionals is primarily cultural; there is suspicion of those from outside the community's own group, particularly those whose technical training is identified with the non-Indian culture.

40

We are now contemplating a broad study of a large number of communities in Guatemala, to learn where people wish to go when they are sick. It can then be determined which type of health care delivery system best fits the patient's needs and demands. If the majority feel they are best "cared for" by a health promoter or empiric of their own culture rather than by professionals of another culture, then those involved with health planning are wasting their time and valuable resources by demanding that only the highly schooled should offer services. If the majority prefer care by health promoters, then it will be reasonable to upgrade the unsophisticated and cease to emphasize the sophisticated. Our guess is that this is true in many areas of the world, regardless of cultural variations. What is needed is to determine what the patient really wants and then take him as an equal partner in the decision-making as to his care and cure.

In addition to the curing aspects of their labours, the health promoters have an impact on public health and nutrition. Our promoters are community catalysts. They work in many spheres other than curative medicine. Vaccinations, tuberculosis control and treatment, literacy programmes, family planning, the organization of men's and women's clubs, agricultural extension, the introduction of fertilizers, new crops and better seeds, chicken projects, improving animal husbandry—all are part of the promoters' work and responsibility.

It may be asked how a promoter can find the time and the talent to be such a community catalyst and be engaged in such a wide variety of community activities. During the training period, which, as mentioned earlier, is continuous, with the promoters trained more than 8 years ago still attending regularly, they are taught expertise in total community concern and involvement. Not only does our medical staff in Chimaltenango participate in the training of the promoters but the programme's agronomist (who is a Guatemalan Indian), family planning workers, visiting government experts, and Peace Corps volunteers add to this diversified training with demonstrations, field visits, and formal classes. Less than half of the time of the training schedule is spent on curative medicine, the remainder being devoted to instruction in total community service.

It may be asked why the promoters are willing to spend so much of their time in non-profit-making work such as their other community service. Besides the profit motive that is involved in their curative work, there is a real dedication to being useful to others in the community, which involves working 7 days a week. This can be explained partly by the nature of the value system of the Guatemalan Indian. Generally, Indians hold respect, dignity, and honesty in high regard. In such a situation self-respect is quite natural and from it there easily follows respect for others and the ability to be genuinely concerned for others in the community. No doubt the prestige gained by being a community leader and community server is also important in motivating these workers to give up so much of their time on behalf of the community.

The best supervision is continued education and training. Supervision includes regular attendance at training sessions, a written and oral examination once monthly, the submission of monthly reports on patients treated and review of their medical records, and field visits by the supervisor to the promoter's treatment centre. If the promoter does not maintain acceptable standards of care and treatment, the medicine cooperative may refuse to sell him medicine.

The profit motive naturally plays a part in the promoters' attitudes towards their jobs. The Cakchiquels are skilled traders with an acute business sense and the idea of a "medical business" dovetails nicely with their concepts. Although it is not encouraged, some promoters make their entire livelihood from their medical practice. Others use it as a supplement. Some have advanced to the point of owning motorcycles so they can reach distant areas more easily. Without exception, every promoter is more secure financially than he was before training; at the same time he renders a service never before performed in his village. Moreover, no promoter receives any pay from the parent organization in Chimaltenango.

The total programme comprises an intensive medical and agricultural extension service that includes Indian agronomists and nurses (these nurses are not graduates but locally trained in our facilities), who make a considerable contribution to the community health promoter programme, working side by side with the promoters and sharing their experience and expertise. For example, when making their field visits, the agronomists and nurses spend time with the local promoter, counselling him and giving other on-the-spot help.

Each of our promoters treats an average of over 1000 patients in a year. The outside cost of the service has been negligible. The expenses involved in training, continued education and supervision are the salary of the one Indian supervisor (US$100 a month), the salary of a Peace Corps volunteer, the time given by the doctor, and a very small amount for training materials. While in training the promoters pay their own expenses. We paid for their bus travel early in the programme but have since discontinued this arrangement. All the remaining funds come from the people in the communities being served on a fee basis. The total outside cost of maintaining the programme for 70 promoters is far less than the cost of training one sophisticated doctor. We estimate our overhead costs at about US$70 a year per promoter, as compared to the US$7500–20 000 required annually to sustain a professional doctor.

We can see no reasons, other than the objections of monopoly and special interest concerns, why a system similar to ours could not be initiated in the developed countries, including the USA. The professional journals and the mass media in general provide ample data on the lack of medical curing by the professionals and on the need for more medical students and more medical schools and classes, for the use of computer analysis, for orientation to rural and slum areas, for emphasis on community medicine, and for obligatory service in deprived areas by medical students and recent graduates. However, these are only balm for the problem. Radical surgery, not sticking plaster, is needed on the medical care delivery system. The entire professional system needs restructuring so that general medical knowledge and simple medical tools are made available to the hundreds of millions of people with the ability to cure themselves. Lest we doctors forget, nature cures most ailments, sometimes in spite of the physician. The majority of medical problems are self-limited and run their natural course. The physician and the profession have usually taken credit for nature's work and have given the impression that the doctor of medicine is responsible for health. However, examination of the causes and natural course of disease reveals that this is a misconception and that the doctor has little to do with the overall health of the population. Many in the profession still cling to the notion that they are curative deities; they have denied, or failed to understand, their stark limitations as real healers. This has led the doctor to be miserly with his information and forced the patient to come to the monopoly for any and all ailments. However, we suspect that this deception and the associated monopolization of medical practice may soon come to an end. We think that during the next half-century medicine will cross the greatest watershed in its history. The doctor of the future will cease to be just a "curer", but will enter his rightful place as a real healer who teaches his patients to care for themselves and to come to him only when the situation is such that nature itself cannot cure and expert, sophisticated help is needed.

Extension services—public health

Except for the training of promoters, our medical extension programme has not developed as we should like, chiefly because of a shortage of time, funds, and trained personnel. Nevertheless, we have moved into this area with considerable energy. Extension work has included the training of intelligent Indian women, known as extension workers, who travel to various villages to work with families and groups to encourage and demonstrate many aspects of community health. This programme consists of such activities as nutrition and hygiene classes, sewing classes, home demonstrations, home gardens, and chicken projects.

The following short narrative illustrates the work of our extension programme. Maria, one of our Indian extension nurses, is working with the women in La Bola de Oro, a village abysmally deprived, with malnutrition, low agricultural production, unjust land tenure, lost hope, and general deprivation as intolerable as can be imagined. When a group of villagers was organized, they expressed interest in activities such as cooking classes, family gardening, obtaining cleaner water, and learning to read a little. But high on their list of priorities was learning to embroider, something unknown to the women even though the finest hand-loom weaving had been done in the village for centuries. Nutrition classes were acceptable, but the women really wanted to embroider, so Maria is teaching them to embroider. Many might say that this is a waste of time and energy, and poor stewardship of funds. Maria says that while the embroidering is going on she enters into various dialogues with the women to get them to consider their other needs carefully. Then the decisions and requests will come from them, will have roots, and will eventually bring meaningful action and results.

Action and results have actually already been achieved to a significant degree in that the women have started a chicken project and a programme of weaving to earn money, garden projects are in operation, and their husbands have also become involved in organizing pig and goat projects and forming a cooperative group to buy a piece of land.

This story illustrates that what may at first sight seem a useless activity with the people can lead to meaningful action if properly dedicated and oriented.

Since these extensionists are Indian women, speak the Cakchiquel language, wear the native garb, and are identified as Indians, they have been a potent force for communication. When not travelling to the country, they work in the clinic and hospital and are always valuable cultural bridges between us and the many Indian patients who come daily for treatment.

The Indian culture in Guatemala is a biophilic one, dedicated to life, family, God, crops, and the earth. It does not take readily to limiting life and family. We sensed this early and we once thought that birth control would not be acceptable in the highlands. However, with the passage of time and more intensive thinking with the people, it became apparent that the Indian's dedication to life can, and does, include family planning. There is an awareness that, although the number of members of their race is an important consideration, proper land use and health, particularly of the children, are related to family size and spacing. Again, our initial impression reflects the usual situation where the "developed" think that the "underdeveloped" have no idea of their needs and how to meet them. The Indians do understand that 6, 8 or 10 children in the family will overtax their land and their food supply. They are genuinely interested in planning their families, but strictly on their own terms.

The family planning service is offered exclusively by Indian nurses. No physician enters into the dialogue or decision-making unless the nurse requests him to do so. Our nurses do not bluntly raise the subject of birth control, explaining what can be done with a particular apparatus, pill, or injection. Instead, the nurse first sits down with the family and considers

44

with them their situation and their own view of it, and why they may wish to limit their family. The technicalities are delayed until the family is deeply and fully involved in the decision-making on its own terms. Once a decision is made for family planning, the service is offered. Since the family makes the decision, the drop-out rate is low.

The majority of families prefer the pill as a family planning method, because of the ease of use. Intrauterine loops are encouraged but they are not nearly so widely accepted as the pill, for several reasons. Inserting a loop involves a vaginal examination, which is only reluctantly accepted by Indian women, even if performed by a nurse of their own culture. Also, there are rumours that the loop causes excessive bleeding and disrupts the normal menstrual cycle. The injectable contraceptives are not encouraged because of the possible serious side effects.

We have made no detailed study of the results of the family planning programme, but do know that there are fewer births per population and more realistic spacing of children, particularly in the areas where more concentrated efforts have been made.

The Indian must be convinced that there will be positive results, not merely the limitation of offspring. The Indian is suspicious of other cultures and their methods. To limit his numbers might lower his level of competitiveness with the *ladinos* (non-Indians). This idea, together with his traditional reliance on his children to carry on when he is too old, makes him somewhat reluctant to limit his family. If he is to be persuaded to consider family planning, he must be assured that those who follow him will have adequate food and land. He knows that half his children die from disease, most of which is linked with malnutrition, and so it must be demonstrated to him that having fewer children can increase survival chances by ensuring better nutrition. So agricultural extension, nutrition advice, and land reform programmes must be integral parts of the family planning concept. While we believe birth control to be important, we must remind readers in the industrial countries that each new Indian child in the Guatemala highlands will use, in his lifetime, only a tiny fraction of the irreplaceable natural resources (iron, aluminium, oil, etc.) that a child born in the USA will use. It requires 25 tons of ore extracted from the earth each year to sustain the average citizen of the USA, as contrasted with a fraction of a ton for the average Indian of Guatemala.

Extension services—agriculture and economics

The typical Indian farmer in the Guatemalan highlands is land-poor. Land holdings are fractioned into tiny plots, since, traditionally, the Indian farmer divides his holdings equally among his sons. However, much of Guatemala is covered by large estates and plantations, often left fallow by their indifferent absentee owners, who maintain titles only because of prestige or family tradition or as a secure investment. Many Indians live on these estates as tenant farmers, owning no land at all.

Faced with such conditions, our extension programme initially concentrated on the obvious approaches—the use of fertilizers, soil and crop improvement, the introduction of better seeds, crop diversification, growing vegetables and cold-weather fruits, chicken projects, veterinary medicine, and other efforts that helped the subsistence farmer to produce more nourishing food for himself and his family. Many of the farmers reached by the programme have increased their yields 2–3 times. In some cases, improvements have been even more dramatic. While the programme has neither time nor money for evaluation, it is obvious to us that health has improved greatly in the areas most affected by our agricultural projects, since much of the disease was related to poor resistance caused by malnutrition.

These efforts, however, have their limitations. One must, of course, respect cultural preferences and do so willingly. One example is maize, a crop almost sacred to the Cakchiquel Indian. Even if he grows nothing else, he always grows maize, consuming it as his staple diet. It would be futile to try to persuade the Cakchiquel to eat higher protein food instead of maize. In any case such a change is not necessary. The Indian is ready to grow and consume other food if it is feasible financially. So, rather than disparage the maize tortilla, which is in any case more nutritious than bread made from bleached white flour, the agricultural programme has concentrated on improving maize yields and satisfying the family needs, deferring the planting of other crops. For the long term, the development of a high-lysene corn that can be grown in the Guatemalan highland climate holds much promise.

Our programme remains flexible with respect to the use of manufactured agricultural accessories. Chemical fertilizers in particular strongly tempt us. Mechanical implements, such as tractors, are less attractive because of the rugged terrain and the cost of buying and maintaining machinery. The programme has employed chemical fertilizers, but only after analysis of soil samples. The fertilizers have definitely improved yields, but now, in view of the rapid rise in price and the worldwide shortage of fertilizers, we have been reminded once again of the hazards entailed by a development programme that relies on outside technology. Just as the medical approach must emphasize disease prevention, releasing people from dependence upon manufactured pharmaceuticals, so must the agricultural phase stress implements that the people can produce themselves. So the programme has now begun experimentation with efficient ways of producing natural fertilizers that control the balance of the basic chemical elements.

The extension agronomists have received their training either with the local government agricultural extension programme or within our own programme, that training being offered by more senior agronomists or Peace Corps volunteers.

Another limitation on the programme is the poverty of the average small farmer. He simply does not have the money to invest in new methods that he considers risky. He finds loans extremely difficult to obtain, and when he does get a loan it is usually from a private money-lender who charges intolerable interest. To meet this need, the programme set up a revolving loan fund to provide farmers with credit on easy terms for specific agricultural projects. Gradually this revolving loan fund is being replaced by a local agricultural and savings and loan cooperative. This cooperative is growing rapidly and already includes many of the people involved in our other programmes. The people themselves manage and control it.

The financing of the project

It may be asked how the medical and agriculture extension workers are paid and how such a programme can be locally self-sustaining. Currently, funds for this extension programme come from out-of-country foundations. We are, however, gradually working towards local funding, using the accumulated interest from our various loan programmes. Interest is charged on land and agricultural loans and as these programmes grow the returning interest will be sufficient to pay the salaries of the various extension workers, thus making outside funding unnecessary. Also, we have a long-term plan that involves a local agricultural and savings and loan cooperative, mentioned above, with which we work very closely. This cooperative, called El Quetzal-Katoki, is rapidly expanding and currently has more than 2000 local members, all Indian. The services of this cooperative include the sale of agricultural supplies and the provision of loans for agricultural investment (not including land loans, which are covered by the "ULEU" programme discussed later). Their last inventory showed that their capital exceeded US$200 000. The interest on the capital enables this large cooperative to make its programme self-sustaining. We have entered into a dialogue with the board of directors of this cooperative and drawn up tentative plans for uniting our total programme with the cooperative, which under this new association will be capable of offering total community services. A family or farmer will then have available to them anything they might need, whether it be a curative medical service, family planning, land and fertilizer loans, agricultural advice, or any other need that might arise—all from local funds, with no outside financial assistance.

In areas of the world where out-of-country sources of funds are not readily available for starting and maintaining community programmes, extension programmes, and loan projects, it may be possible to interest local government in making funds available as grants or loans or to obtain money from the private sector for rural investment. Each area has its unique situation, which it must evaluate in terms of culture, economy, tradition, and local realities.

The lack of land to farm remains the most formidable obstacle to success of our agricultural programmes. Indeed, land hunger is the source of almost every major problem in these Indian highlands. Since enormous numbers of farmers own no land or own a piece so small that it is insufficient for family needs (even with our improved techniques), the majority of up-land Indians are forced to migrate seasonally to the tropical coffee and cotton plantations on the Pacific slopes. There, they receive low wages and live in squalid conditions. This aggravates the primary health problems of infectious disease and malnutrition and also absorbs the time that the farmer otherwise would spend on improving crop yields in his own highland village. Furthermore, when the farmer does not own, or control through collectives, a suitable piece of land in the highlands, he has scant incentive to improve the land. If he were to improve the soil by taking extensive conservative measures such as building terraces and contour ditches, or by applying fertilizer and using a simple plough, the value of the land would rise and the owner would demand more rent—and even then might not let the land to the same farmer. As a result, many Indian farmers refuse to employ techniques that they know will improve land and crops.

Responding to this dire need, a new programme is being established to provide loans to communities of farmers who wish to buy their own land. Loans are made only to groups, so that communal farms will be encouraged, the cost of extension services reduced, and the purchase of larger properties made possible. The greater the amount of land being purchased the better the bargaining position of the buyer. The revolving loan fund programme is called "ULEU", which means "land" in Cakchiquel, and is governed by a board of directors, who are the extensionists and the representatives of the cooperatives, all local people. The loans are long-term with low interest rates by Guatemalan standards. The farmers do their own nego-tiating with the landlords to determine a sale price and then choose one of two or three payment plans. The response already obtained from groups of farmers has been much greater than the programme can handle financially at this time.

We by no means suggest that this approach is the ideal structure for land reform, but it is a good option for a voluntary programme that wishes to present a show-case demonstration project. We hope to show that land reform can be effective if it is embraced by a complex of community services as well as those primarily agricultural. We also hope to demonstrate how closely land reform is tied to public health. We, as sophisticated physicians, might not have seen the connexion ourselves if the Cakchiquel people had not pointed it out to us. We who work in development are always indebted to the people who teach us through their own responsiveness.

Our 12 years in Guatemala among these natural, loving, responsive, and industrious people, our friends the Cakchiquels, have wrought a major change in our perceptions. We came to cure the sick. Now we stay to help cure the basic causes of sickness.

The reproducibility of the programme

It is often asked whether the programme can be reproduced elsewhere, in Guatemala or in other countries. In Guatemala, the Government has gone beyond the mere authorization of our community health promoter programme and has used it as a model for setting up the health training programme in the Ministry of Health, and, in fact, we were asked to help in the training of some of the supervisors and trainers for this Government programme. Whether the programme could be used outside Guatemala would depend on numerous factors such as possible local interference in this type of programme by the local medical professionals, whether the government agrees with the idea of alternative health services being offered, whether the people accept such alternatives, and various other local situations. We know that in many countries those in both national and local authority are seeking alternatives, recognizing that by no stretch of the imagination can medical professionals really "care" for all the people in need, particularly in the developing world with its large populations and limited resources.

Guidelines for the public health of the rural poor

— In poor areas of the world, as elsewhere, medicine must be practised for the benefit of the patient, not for the convenience and welfare of the doctor. Public health work should begin with a dialogue with the people, encouraging them to consider themselves and their situation and to state their needs. People everywhere have their own ideas about what should be done with their lives, health, and homes. The effective professional listens before he acts, treats his patients as an equal in decision-making, and does not force his own ideas and standards on those he serves.
— A programme that relies too heavily on outside technical and financial assistance is destined for trouble. Almost any technically trained person, regardless of nationality, is considered an outsider in the vast areas inhabited by the rural poor. In many countries there are distinct racial, cultural, and linguistic groupings carrying economic, political, and class implications. In addition, there is an enormous difference in outlook between the urbanized technician and the rural poor. The technician is usually assured of a physically comfortable existence while the poor person

often struggles to exist from day to day. This discrepancy alone accounts for enormous differences in perception. The poor man is no fool and he must be thoroughly convinced that the technocrat's arguments are valid before he will risk deviation from age-tested patterns of living, especially if he has to pay for the change.

— Nationalism is perhaps one of the most difficult problems facing innovators in a developing country. Most native professionals are as alien and suspect to the rural poor as the foreign professionals, separated from the people as they often are by formidable racial, linguistic, and cultural barriers. National professionals, whether they be priest, preacher, doctor, or engineer, can exert much more influence over their own people than foreigners can. These professionals are often quick to adopt nationalist attitudes when they find their own power, prestige, and privileges threatened by a popular programme—particularly one initiated by foreigners. The greatest challenge to such a programme is how to achieve acceptability in the eyes of the national elite without being stifled by the professional bureaucracies. Control of a programme should be vested in the people the programme is designed to serve and should never be dominated by the aristocrats.

— Beware of the cry for "higher standards". Professionals love to boost "standards" for any programme, thereby driving up the cost of equipment and expertise and putting the programme beyond the reach of a humble community. Quality should never be equated with high cost. Unfortunately, the medical profession has waged an extensive propaganda campaign in this direction. They would have us believe, for instance, that expensive open-heart surgery is the pinnacle of accomplishment in medicine. However, in three-quarters of the world, disease that could be easily and inexpensively treated runs rampant. If the medical profession declines to tackle the basic ailments that it already knows how to treat and prevent, then it is not entitled to indulge in extravagantly expensive techniques for the rich few.

— A public health programme aimed exclusively at curing the sick will have little effect on the health of the rural poor. A programme that includes preventive medicine, nutrition, and hygiene will fare somewhat better, but it too will fail to do the job. A programme expanded by family planning and earnest work on increasing crop yields on the family farm will accomplish more. However, a programme that fails to deal with the fundamental problem—ownership of the land—will meet with no more than modest success.

— The truly successful public health programme among the rural poor must tackle basic problems of economic and political development. This by no means indicates that programme leaders should plunge into controversial national issues or ally themselves with specific political movements. A programme must be detached from factional politics if it is to respond to the people without power. Yet, there are levels below those of national politics where the people can learn to control their own lives through politics and economics. A cooperative is a good example, since it responds to financial need and builds local leadership. The cooperative is no panacea, but it is often a practical move in the right direction, laying a foundation for people power in the politics of survival.

— The stronger the orientation toward those being served, the more successful the programme is likely to be. The essential first steps are: listen to the people, appreciate them, love them, take them into your confidence, and try to be at one with them.

— Avoid offering service on your terms only. If you do a demographic survey, be sure that it includes the questions, "What do *you* think your needs are ?" and "How do *you* think we can help you ?".

— Local community health committees should be organized and functioning before the first aspirin or dressing is handed out. The committees should then select the people to be trained to offer service, supervise them, discipline them, report on them, and control them. Committees should set the standards of service and the prices to be charged.

— The outside help needed in materials, manpower, direction, and supervision should always conform to local custom and tradition. The technician or physician should dedicate himself to training local counterparts as quickly as possible.

— Training programmes should permit trainees to continue their usual work, family, and community relationships, with absence from home kept to a minimum. Training programmes at distant centres often disrupt family and community links and may corrupt the trainee by exposure to a foreign culture and life style that makes return to his community difficult and sometimes impossible.

— Medical training demands the use of clinical teaching on patients in either a dispensary or hospital, so that the clinical picture is clearly seen, appreciated, and understood.

— The treatment of ailments should be according to symptoms, not diagnosis. Even people with sophisticated schooling often misinterpret symptoms when making a diagnosis. Our experience is that symptom treatment results in relatively low error, considering that most medical problems are simple and, in the natural course of events, heal themselves.

— Trainees must be taught what not to treat as well as what to treat and how. The future of non-professional curing demands that this concept should not be violated.

— The supervision and continued education of lay curers is essential, the nature of the supervision depending on local conditions. We require regular attendance at clinical training sessions, regular examinations, regular visits by the supervisor to the health promoter's home, and regular reports from local community health committees on the calibre of the health promoter's work, its acceptance, and the range of fees charged.

— The fees should be decided locally, and the central agency should never put anyone on the payroll. The community being served pays—with no exceptions. The only people on the central payroll should be the trainers and supervisors, and no one else. Curative medical services should pay for themselves. In a total programme income should cover all costs, with the proviso that since certain individuals cannot pay at the time of treatment a credit system must be introduced, with generous use of the "Robin Hood" principle, namely, charging higher fees to those who can afford to pay and asking considerably lower fees from the genuinely poor.

— Dependence on outside finances saps local responsibility and may jeopardize the supply of services and materials.

— Health has many facets—economic, political and social. Each must be taken into account when the epidemiology of any human health problem is being considered. Proper care for any ailment—physical or social—demands dedication to the treatment of causes, not merely the amelioration of current pain.

CHINA: Health station, Sing Sing Production Brigade. Kao Ning-shin, the brigade midwife, is seen on the right.

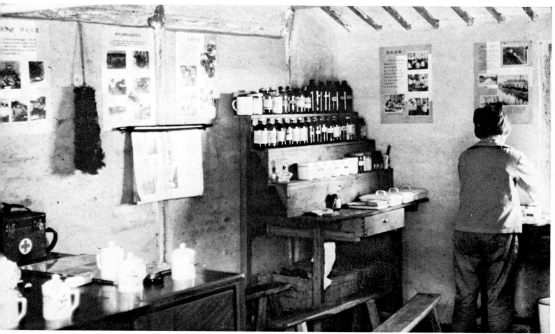

CHINA: A doctor of "Western" medicine (left) and a doctor of traditional Chinese medicine (back to camera) in a hypertension clinic in Shanghai.

CHINA: The barefoot doctor at Tachai Brigade health station chopping herbs to make medicines.

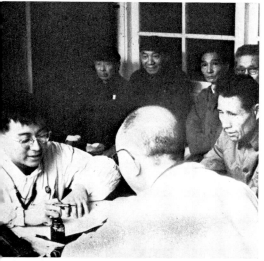

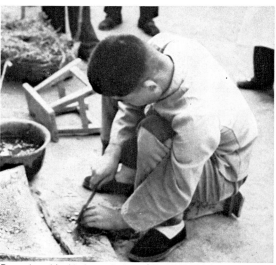

CUBA: A rural hospital and doctor's living quarters in a mountainous district of Oriente. In such districts, hospitals of 10-30 beds are the basic unit of the rural health area.

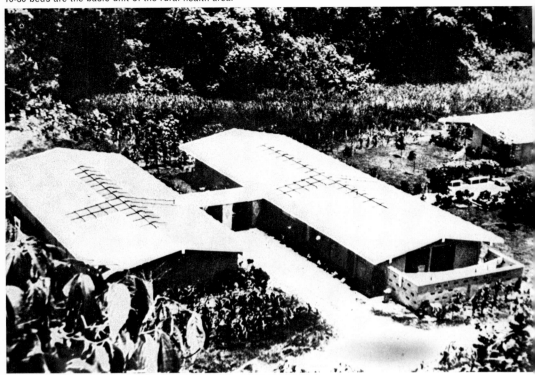

Reproduced by kind permission of the Ministry of Health, Cuba

CUBA: The person responsible for health in a Committee for the Defence of the Revolution administers oral polio-myelitis vaccine to a child in his block.

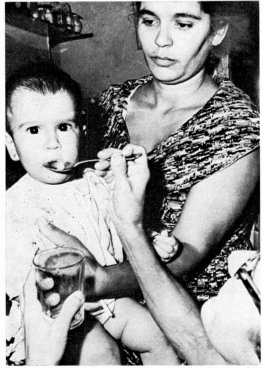

Reproduced by kind permission of the Ministry of Health, Cuba

GUATEMALA: Daniel Cujcuy, president of the Quetz Katoki Cooperative, explaining the programme to a group farmers.

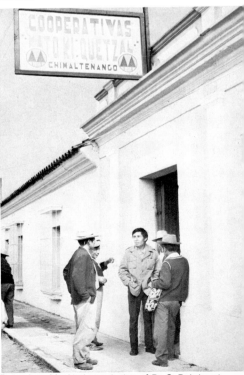

Reproduced by kind permission of Dr C. Behrhorst

GUATEMALA: Supervisor Carlos Xocquic taking a class for community health promoters.

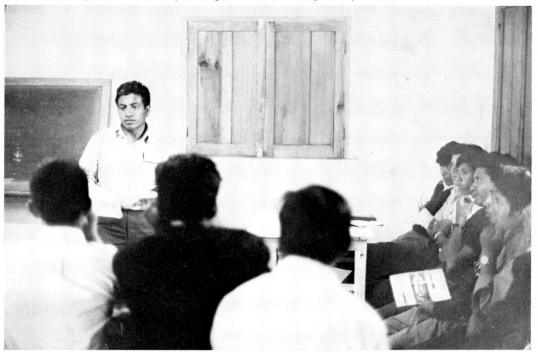

Reproduced by kind permission of Dr C. Behrhorst

INDIA: A village health worker giving health education.

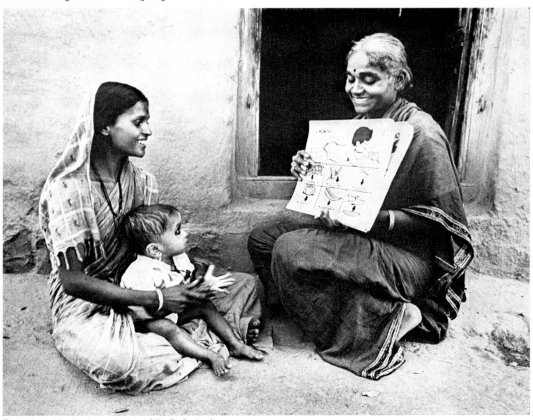

Reproduced by kind permission of Dr R. S. Arole

INDIA: A health education stall in a market place.

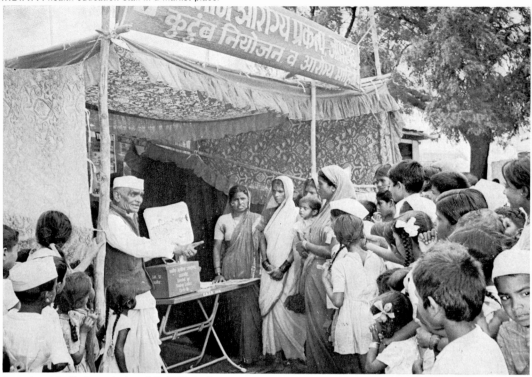

Reproduced by kind permission of Dr R. S. Arole

INDIA: A patient arriving in an ox cart at the main centre, Jamkhed.

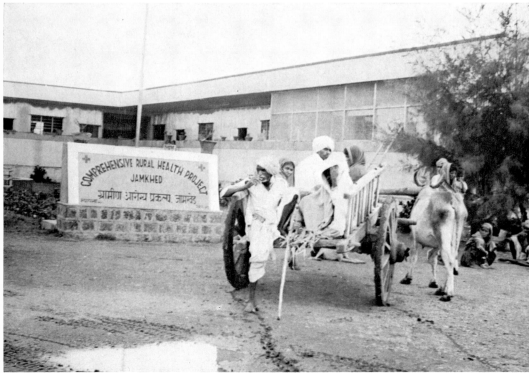

Reproduced by kind permission of Dr R. S. Arole

INDONESIA: The goat cooperative.

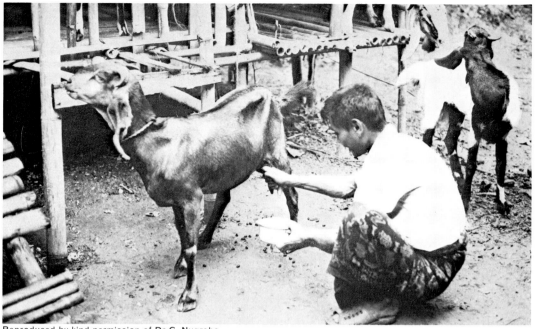

Reproduced by kind permission of Dr G. Nugroho

(RIGHT) INDONESIA: The mini-dam in Sirkandi (Klampok).
Reproduced by kind permission of Dr G. Nugroho

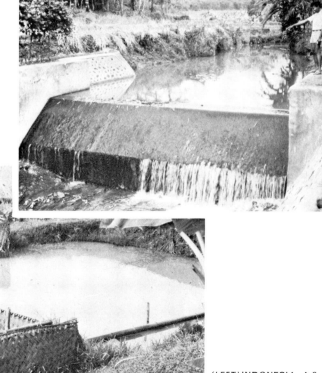

(LEFT) INDONESIA: A fish pond in Sirkandi (Klampok).
Reproduced by kind permission of Dr G. Nugroho

IRAN: A *behdasht yar* (male health worker) supervising the building of latrines.

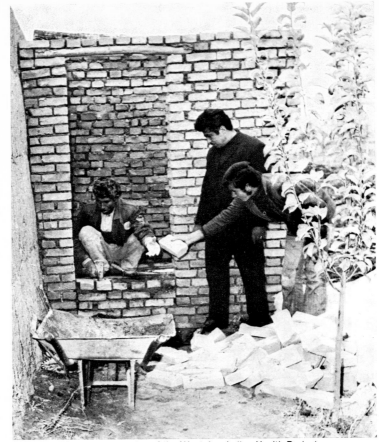

Reproduced by kind permission of the West Azerbaijan Health Project

IRAN: A *behyar mama rustai* (rural nurse/midwife) on a home visit.

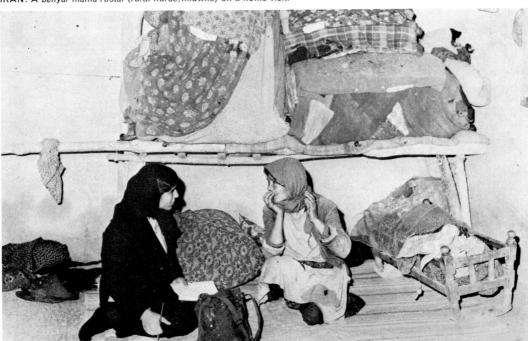

Reproduced by kind permission of the West Azerbaijan Health Project

NIGER: A nurse checking a village pharmacy in the presence of two village health workers.

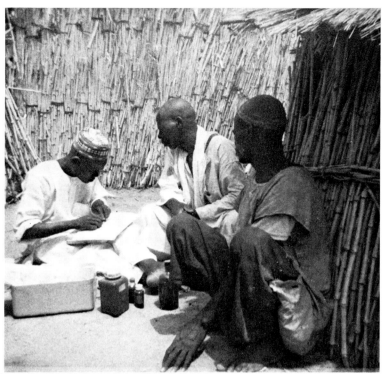

Reproduced by kind permission of Dr G. Fournier

TANZANIA: A class of rural medical aides in progress.

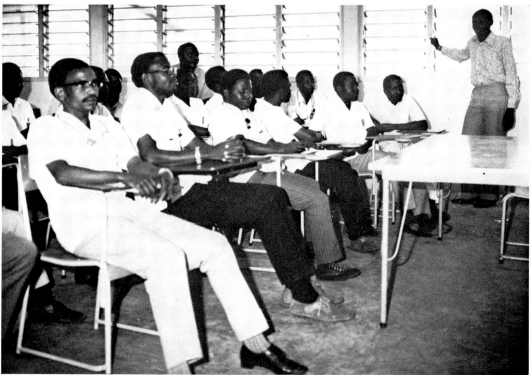

Reproduced by kind permission of Tanzania Information Services

TANZANIA: A rural self-help project — digging a trench for a rural water supply.

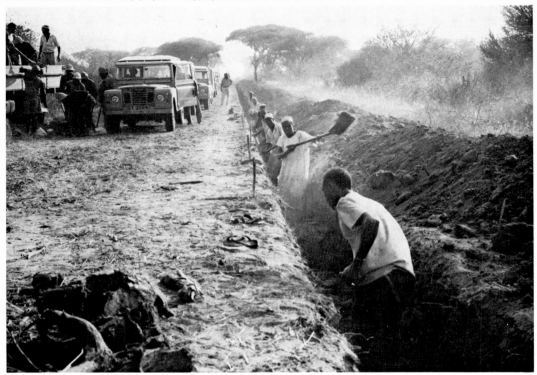

Reproduced by kind permission of Tanzania Information Services

VENEZUELA: The auxiliary is taking the temperature of a child brought by its mother with an acute febrile condition, cough and dyspnoea. The child received treatment (including penicillin injection) at the dispensary and recovered.

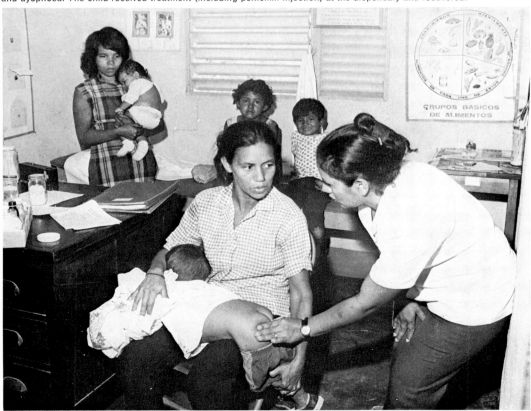

Reproduced by kind permission of the Ministry of Health and Social Security, Venezuela

VENEZUELA: The auxiliary has to find her way to the most isolated homes, often through difficult terrain. The only way of reaching Laguna village (1682 inhabitants), on Lake Maracaibo, is by boat.

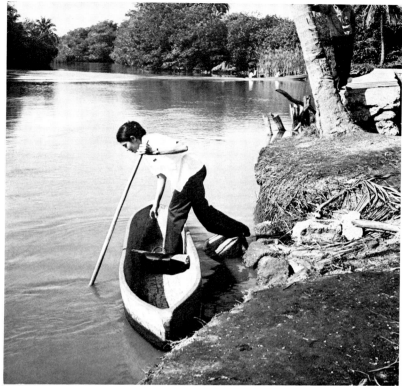

WHO photograph (P. Almasy)

VENEZUELA: Señor Luis Angel Pricto is the auxiliary in the small village of Guavera. On learning that a farmer has been visited by a member of his family coming from a region where there was a smallpox epidemic, he comes to vaccinate the whole family.

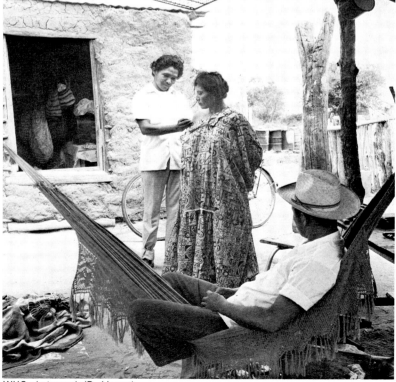

WHO photograph (P. Almasy)

No. 6

Referencia para la Médicatura Rural u Hospital

El Dispensario: _Bethil Municipio Biruaca_____

Refiere a: _____

A la Medicatura Rural u Hospital para su tratamiento.

Se le dió los "Primeros Auxilios siguientes"

_Segalta Jose Ubaldme de 12 años de edad tiene
5 días de enfermo con fiebre vomito I dolor del
ombligo al lado derecho I de malle de la misma
pierna, no le apliqui tratamiento lo envio a ese
inmediatamente_

Fecha _4-12-63_   _Julia Saurs_
                                  Firma de la Auxiliar

VENEZUELA: This is a reproduction of a referral form filled in by an auxiliary to refer the case to the nearest centre. With this referral form, which was written in a simple way but clearly stated the main symptoms, the patient was taken by a relative to the nearest hospital, where a diagnosis of acute appendicitis was made and a surgical operation immediately performed. The patient recovered. The following is a translation of the referral form:

Referral to *medicatura rural* or hospital   No. 6

Dispensary: Bethel, Municipio Biruaca

Refers:

to the *medicatura rural* or hospital for treatment.

The following first-aid care was given:

... (patient's name) of 12 years of age has been sick for 5 days with fever, vomiting, fainting, and pain in the umbilicus on the right side, causing weakness of the leg on the same side. I did not give any treatment but sent him to you immediately.

(date)   (auxiliary's signature)

Reproduced by kind permission of the Ministry of Health and Social Security, Venezuela.

THE AYURVEDIC SYSTEM OF MEDICINE IN INDIA

K. N. UDUPA [a]

Medicine has evolved in three phases—magic, religion, and science. Throughout the ages, man has devised ways and means of caring for the sick in the community depending mainly on the community's notions of the origins and causes of disease.

Until the discovery of bacteria, many communicable diseases were attributed to supernatural causes and regarded as evidence of the displeasure of ancestral gods and evil spirits, or to black magic. Such beliefs are still held by many less sophisticated communities in developing countries and indigenous healers therefore undertake elaborate exorcising rituals on behalf of the sick and mentally afflicted. Among such communities, diseases have been classified into three broad categories—those curable by indigenous medicine, those curable by modern medicine, and those that are self-limiting and not affected by either system.

There is therefore no vacuum anywhere in regard to health care, but such care, though psychologically supportive to the individual, may be largely ineffective or even harmful through lack of medical and scientific knowledge, skills, and technical resources. However, certain aspects of the classical clinical approach to modern scientific medicine, particularly in the developing countries, are in some respects biased, incomplete and, indeed, potentially harmful to some communities because of missing sociocultural factors.

In this respect, the great traditions of Arabic, Chinese, and Indian medicine are important, particularly in relation to the emergence of scientific medicine in the 19th and 20th centuries. An analysis of these traditions is needed for medical sociology and is relevant to the practical problem of improving health care, and in particular following a decision to effect total health care coverage for a particular population group.

In 1946 the Government of India set up a committee to study indigenous systems of medicine in India and its report was published in 1948. The inquiry was concerned with the history of Ayurveda, or Hindu medicine

[a] In collaboration with R. H. O. Bannerman, Division of Health Manpower Development, World Health Organization, Geneva, Switzerland.

(including Sidha), and of the Unani Tibbi indigenous systems of medicine and their place in India today.

Ayurveda is reputed to have been practised for over 3000 years, its history being divided into four periods: (1) the Vedic period, (2) the original research and classical periods, (3) a period of compilation of Ayurvedic methods and periods of Rasa Tantras and Sidhas—chemist physicians, and (4) a period of stagnation and eventually recompilation. Ayurveda was at its height during the second and third periods. There were treatises on general medicine, anatomy, gynaecology, obstetrics (including Caesarean section and destructive operations on the fetus), and surgery (including lithotomy and rhinoplasty). Anatomical dissections were undertaken. Persons suffering from infectious diseases were isolated. Immunity was known to the ancient Hindus and inhalation anaesthesia was also used. The principles of dietetics were well appreciated and utilized in the care of the sick.

At the beginning of the Christian era, Ayurveda had spread far and wide and had influenced the systems of medicine in Egypt, Greece, Rome, and Arabia. Surgery, including the couching of cataracts and bone-setting, was practised and the surgery of those wounded in battle was well established. The advent of Moslem rule brought with it the Unani or Arabic system of practice, and both were utilized in India for the benefit of the people. The introduction of Western European surgery followed British rule in India and this tended to weaken the influence of Ayurvedic practice. By the end of the 19th century the indigenous systems had become static and their practice had largely fallen into the hands of untrained persons without the competence to practise Ayurvedic medicine.

The report stated that, although both the Ayurvedic and Unani systems had become static, further investigation of these systems might lead to many valuable contributions to modern medical science.

In 1827, classes in Ayurvedic medicine were begun at the Government Sanskrit College, Calcutta. These classes were discontinued in 1835 and the Calcutta Medical College of Western Medicine was established. As with the colonial medical service in its formative years, the training and services provided were designed essentially for the expatriate ruling community. This engendered a reaction, particularly among Indian nationalists, and following sporadic attempts at rehabilitation of the Ayurvedic and Unani systems, provincial governments showed interest in their revival. In 1920 the Indian National Congress passed a resolution to the effect that, having regard to the widely prevalent and generally accepted utility of the Ayurvedic and Unani systems of medicine in India, earnest efforts should be made by the people of India to popularize schools, colleges, and hospitals for instruction and treatment in accordance with these indigenous systems.

Some provincial and state governments interested themselves in the use of Indian medicine for rural medical relief. Schools and colleges of Indian medicine were opened in Madras, Bombay, Delhi, Bengal, and other states to train competent practitioners of Indian medicine with a good working knowledge of modern medicine so that they could render comprehensive medical service to the rural population. Proposals were put forward to promote research and eventually to integrate the Indian and the modern scientific systems. In the report it was recommended that health teams should include doctors, physical training experts, sanitarians, physiotherapists, nurses, and midwives.

The Committee expressed the view that, as all different systems—Ayurveda, Unani, modern scientific medicine, homeopathy, etc.—have the prime objectives of maintaining health and preventing and curing disease, they should all be properly investigated for the benefit of humanity and integrated into a single health care system. Separate systems of Indian and modern medicine were not envisaged in the report, although the available information indicated that Indian medicine, though relatively static, still gave medical relief to over 80% of the population.

As a result of recommendations of the 1948 and subsequent committees, the Central Council of Indian Medicine was constituted by the Government of India in 1971. The Council's main functions include (*a*) the recognition of qualifications in Indian medicine, (*b*) the prescription of minimum standards of education in Indian medicine, and (*c*) the maintenance of a central register of practitioners. The Council has worked quickly and has already established minimum standards of undergraduate education and introduced a curriculum for adoption by the college of Indian medicine. Minimum standards and curricula for postgraduate education have also been established.

The science and philosophy of Ayurvedic medicine

The ancient method of study

The system of ancient Indian medicine—Ayurveda—was developed against the rich background of social, cultural, and philosophical principles prevailing in India between the period 600 B.C. to A.D. 700. The three great authors Charaka, Sushruta, and Vagbhata were much influenced by the Sankhya and Yoga philosophies of that time. In addition, they followed the scientific methods of study that were then in existence. These methods were (1) direct perception through one of the sense organs, (2) inference, (3) revelations after intense observations, and (4) common sense (the laws of probability). A few of the statements in Ayurveda were supported by scientific proof and these can now be verified by modern scientific methods. Other statements appear to be purely abstract, without scientific proof, and these may be regarded as philosophical speculations that cannot be tested by the currently available modern scientific methods.

These authors discussed in great detail not only the bodily illnesses but also the different psychosomatic problems during health and disease. The philosophy of Ayurveda can help us to understand the different psychosomatic disorders occurring in man and also the methods they adopted to manage them.

Basic elements

According to the principles of Ayurveda, the human being is a miniature imitation of the universe. Whatever properties are contained in the universe are also found in the human body and whatever are in the human body are found in the universe. According to Indian philosophy, the universe consists of five gross elements—earth, water, fire, air, and the ethereal parts of the sky—and the same factors constitute the basic elements of the human body. However, in a human body, life does not depend only on these five bodily components but also on the presence of normally functioning sense organs, and of the mind and the soul. Thus Sushruta defined the healthy person as follows: "He is the healthy man who possesses the balance of body humours, proper functioning of all the body elements and who has the pleasant disposition of mind, soul, and sense organs". Therefore, according to Ayurveda, if one wants to study medicine one has to understand man as a whole and appreciate his psychosomatic constitution.

Since the middle of the 19th century, these humoral theories have been completely discarded and replaced, in modern medical sciences, by cell biology and human physiology. However, humoral theories are occasionally invoked to explain certain physiological activities, for example, the neurohumours such as acetylcholine, catecholamine, histamine, and serotonin. The three humours recognized in Ayurveda—Vata, Pitha, and Kapha—can be compared with the modern neurohumours acetylcholine, catecholamine, and histamine, respectively. All the theories and practice of Ayurveda can easily be explained scientifically on the basis of these three humours of Ayurveda.

According to Ayurveda, all bodily structures and functions are controlled by these three humours. In each individual one of the three humours is predominant, thus giving rise to a specific type of psychosomatic constitution. Human beings inherit the body constitution genetically from their parents, and, depending upon the predominance of a particular humour at the time of conception, have a predominance of one humour in the body. Though the body constitution can be influenced to a certain extent by the physical and psychological environment, it remains essentially the same throughout the individual's lifetime.

In Ayurveda, three main types of body constitution have been described, depending upon the predominance of the humours—Vata, Pitha, and Kapha; the three types correspond, respectively, with the ectomorphic, mesomorphic, and endomorphic types of constitution described by Sheldon. In addition to these three main types of body constitution there can be combinations of two humours in one person and also a balance of all three humours in some people, thus bringing the total number of types of body constitution to seven.

The main characteristics of these three main types of body constitution described in Ayurveda are as follows:

Vata constitution (ectomorphic, neurotropic, or acetylcholine-predominant): a person with this constitution usually has a thin body and a very labile temperament. He normally develops a quick response to a stimulus and frequently moves his eyes, jaws, tongue, head, shoulders, hands, and feet without any definite purpose. He is very talkative and is quickly affected by fear, anger, likes and dislikes, and by good and bad. He is quick to grasp and also to forget facts. The hair on his head, face, and body is thick and rough. He usually has rough nails, teeth, hands, and feet. Such persons are more likely to develop functional disorders such as excessive nervousness, insomnia, and tremors, and also stress disorders such as peptic ulcer, ulcerative colitis, etc.

Pitha constitution (mesomorphic, or catecholamine-predominant): a person with this constitution has a moderately well-built muscular body and is courageous and strong. He eats well and performs physical work diligently. He usually has scanty soft hair on the head, face, and body and develops baldness at an early age. On slight provocation he usually develops symptoms referable to the circulatory system, such as rapid pulse, a sharp rise in blood pressure, palpitations, or other cardiac symptoms. These persons are likely, at a relatively early age, to develop, on exposure to stress, hypertension and coronary thrombosis.

Kapha constitution (endomophic, histamine secretors): a person with this constitution usually has a bulky and heavy body with smooth rounded face and limbs. He is usually slow in action and speech. He is also slow in his gait and all his undertakings, and is slow to change in mood. He normally has a good appetite and hence enjoys his meals. He usually becomes susceptible to diabetes mellitus and allergic manifestations such as asthma, rhinitis, and eczema. He is also likely to develop arthritis and fibrositis, which can make him an invalid at a relatively early age. He is not excitable and rarely becomes angry and irritable.

In addition to these three main types of constitution, there can be combinations of two of the types in one person if two of the three humours are predominant. These people will show a mixture of the above qualities depending upon which humour is predominant.

57

People can also be classified according to their psychic constitution. Whereas the constitution of the physical body cannot be changed, man's psychic constitution can be changed by his own efforts, through the practice of Yoga. According to Yoga, the mind is in a continuous state of fluctuation like the waves of the ocean. It is agitated from the outside by the exciting sensory perceptions and from the inside by the memories of emotional factors such as passions, desires, anger, pride, jealousy, and delusion. So long as his mind is agitated and in a state of continuous motion man cannot have peace of mind. The main purpose of the Yogic practice is therefore to calm down agitated minds and minimize the turbulent waves.

According to Ayurveda, the sense organs, or Indriyas, are the main sensory gateways of the body through which the body receives all information from its environment. These sense organs have a vital function to play in giving accurate information about the surroundings to the mind and through it to the soul. They have two parts, the sense organs proper such as eyes, ears, etc., and their corresponding centres in the brain, which enable this information to be stored properly.

The soul, or Atma, or consciousness is the main part and gives life to the body. It does not directly comprehend any object or idea from the world outside and it receives information only through the sense organs and the mind. Thus the capacity for intelligently perceiving the world outside differs from person to person since no two persons have similar types of body, mind, or sense organs. In fact, the life of an individual consists of coordinated activities of all its component parts such as the body, the mind, the sense organs, and the soul. If all these parts function well in a coordinated manner, the person remains healthy. However, when coordination between these components breaks down, individually or collectively, the person becomes ill.

The disease process

According to Ayurveda, illness occurs if there is any derangement in the body humours such as Vata, Pitha, and Kapha, or in the psychic factors such as Satwe, Rajas, and Tamas caused by either excessive or inadequate interactions.

The activity of the three humours of the body may increase or decrease when they are acted upon by various predisposing factors. In the first stage an excess of the humours occurs at their sites of production in different parts of the body. In the second stage the accumulated humours spread in the body. In the third stage they move, alone or jointly, throughout the body and cause the systemic symptoms of the disease. In the fourth stage the humours become localized in some organ or part of the body and after localization produce specific symptoms depending upon the structure and function of the affected organs or tissues. In the fifth stage there is overt manifestation of the disease in a given organ, and in the sixth stage either the disease process resolves in a particular organ or forms an ulcerative lesion through which all the vitiated humours are evacuated. At this stage the entire disease process is usually terminated; otherwise a chronic inflammatory process ensues.

The main purpose of understanding the development of the disease process is to plan appropriate treatment by the elimination process, such as giving emetics or purgatives. Where this is not feasible, the vitiated humours should be neutralized by the process of oxidation or conjugation into relatively non-toxic products, which are then eliminated in the urine or faeces.

In epidemic diseases such as severe smallpox, the constitution of the body is unable to play any part in counteracting the massive infection. Here the disease process is dominant and, in such a state, when the individual body constitution is put out of action, very little individual variation occurs in the process and course of the disease. In fact, there will be some uniformity with regard to clinical features and laboratory findings as is seen in various eruptive fevers. However, in chronic diseases the individual constitution will be able to demonstrate resistance, depending upon its strength, and there will therefore be variation in the presentation and course of the disease.

The practice of Ayurvedic medicine

There is still considerable deficiency in our knowledge with regard to the psychosomatic and stress disorders, which are rapidly becoming more prevalent. As a result, it has not been possible to prevent the growing incidence of such disorders as coronary thrombosis, hypertension, peptic ulcer; nor has it been possible to control them in an effective manner. In fact, some of these disorders are rapidly becoming the main "killers" in modern society. There is, therefore, an obvious need to study these disorders from a different angle, from both the preventive and curative points of view, by making an integrated psychomatic approach as described in Ayurveda.

In Ayurveda, as in modern medicine, there are two major components of medical practice — preventive and curative.

Preventive measures

The preventive aspects of the practice of Ayurveda consist of the following three components: personal and social hygiene, the use of rejuvenating measures to prevent aging and decay, and the practice of Yoga to provide tranquillity of mind and complete physical relaxation.

Personal and social hygiene

In Ayurveda a regulated daily life of getting up early in the morning is recommended with the performance of certain prescribed routines to preserve good physical and mental health. Every day, after evacuating the bowels and cleaning the teeth, the subject should perform Yoga exercises. These are followed by a bath, prayers, regulated diet, and then work, adequate rest, and sleep.

Rejuvenating measures

Two methods are described in Ayurveda for this purpose—"Rasayana", or rejuvenation, and "Vajukarana", or the use of aphrodisiacs (virilizing agents). To achieve both these aims, several drugs and other measures have been described. The main aims of Rasayana are (1) to prevent aging and increase longevity, (2) to improve the memory and intelligence, (3) to increase immunity and body resistance against disease and decay, (4) to give lustre and vitality to the body, and (5) to maintain optimum strength of the body and the sense organs.

There are many well-known herbs that may be given singly or in combination for a prolonged period to provide these desired effects. In addition to the use of drugs, certain exercises and other measures may be carried out to help maintain good bodily and mental health. The various Yoga practices are commonly used for the purpose.

The practice of Yoga

The word "Yoga" means "union" and its exponents claim that by continuous practice of Yoga one can maintain a perfect union of body, mind, and soul, leading to complete tranquillity and peace.

In order to suit the convenience of the individual, a certain selection of Yoga practices should be performed—for example, a few postural exercises, a few breathing exercises, and then some type of meditation. Such a selection of Yoga practices does not take more than 30 minutes and therefore can be done either in the morning or in the evening, as convenient. A selected practice of Yoga should be planned for each individual by an experienced teacher, depending upon the individual's body constitution, temperament, age, and any physical ailments. In a recent study conducted on volunteers who were subjected to various postural and breathing exercises for six months, it was found that there was a significant increase in vital capacity and a decrease in the rate of respiration and heart beat per minute. These volunteers also showed significant decreases in body weight, blood sugar, and blood cholesterol at the end of the six months' experimental period. The rate of urinary excretion of corticosteroids and testosterone was increased. They also demonstrated an improved memory quotient and reduced neuroticism.

The volunteers who practised meditation showed a significant reduction in plasma cortisol, urinary corticosteroids, and urinary nitrogen excretion. At the same time, these volunteers showed significant increases in the blood levels of the different neurohumours and related enzymes. These findings indicate that after meditation the subjects were physically stable and silent, and mentally very active. The practice of Yoga may prove an effective method of keeping fit, both physically and mentally.

In addition, specific Yoga practices have also been used to overcome certain clinical conditions. Thus following the practice of "Shavasana", or the assumption of the posture of the dead for three months, it was noted that 18 out of 21 persons with hypertension had much relief of their symptoms and could either discontinue their antihypertensive drugs or reduce the dosage. Similarly it has been observed that regular practice of Yoga helps patients overcome the early stages of asthma, diabetes mellitus, and thyrotoxicosis.

Curative treatment in Ayurveda

There are four main curative aspects of the practice of Ayurvedic medicine: (1) administration of medicine internally, (2) application of medicinal preparations externally, (3) surgical measures, and (4) treatment by psychosomatic measures.

Internal medicine and therapeutics

The internal administration of drugs plays an important part in treatment. The drugs are used mainly to eliminate the causative factors, including morbid humours, from the body, by causing vomiting or purging, and by the use of different types of enemata and inhalations. These eliminating processes are carried out as far as possible before starting any prolonged curative drug therapy, rejuvenating therapy, or even surgical treatment.

The treatment of rheumatoid arthritis may be taken as an example of treatment according to Ayurvedic principles. Here all the bodily humours become vitiated and settle in the joints, big and small. In order to counteract this process, various eliminating procedures are carried out, these being followed by specific drug therapy, for example, with *gum guggulu* and its preparations.

The second type of treatment is aimed at neutralizing the morbid humours by giving appropriate drugs, diet, and physiotherapy. For this purpose Ayurveda describes a large number of herbal, mineral, and biological preparations to be used singly or in various combinations, depending upon their pharmacodynamic properties. An example of this type of treatment is seen in the management of hemiplegia following a cerebrovascular accident. For such patients Ayurvedic physicians give specific drugs to stimulate regeneration of the peripheral nerves. Purified nux

61

vomica and other drugs with similar properties are given for prolonged periods. The preparations are mostly in the form of powders, liquid extracts, tinctures, decoctions, and tablets. In recent years many attempts have been made to standardize the preparation of these drugs and also to isolate active principles from them. *Rauwolfia serpentina* is one such drug whose active principles have been extensively used all over the world. Many other similar drugs have been investigated in various centres, and no doubt more useful drugs will be discovered in the future.

In addition to drug treatments, Ayurveda attaches great importance to diet. A large variety of dietetic preparations have been found extremely valuable for maintaining the proper nutritional status of patients during their illness. For example, after the onset of acute gastroenteritis in children, modern physicians would advise immediate fluid therapy parenterally. Ayurvedic physicians would, however, try to maintain the fluid balance in these children by carefully planning the oral fluid intake, administering appropriate antiemetic and antidiarrhoeal treatment. They advise the intake of specific fluids such as whey water, boiled rice water, and fresh coconut water. Similarly they recommend specific fruit juices with astringent properties, such as apple juice and pomegranate juice. The intake of milk is forbidden in such cases.

In this way Ayurveda describes treatments for all types of acute and chronic illnesses. The current Ayurvedic treatments appear to be very effective in cases of chronic metabolic diseases such as diabetes mellitus, atherosclerosis, and lipid storage diseases. Similarly, arthritis of various types, different types of gastrointestinal and urinary tract disease, asthma, allergy, some of the specific skin diseases, chronic neurological diseases, and some mental ailments are also amenable to Ayurvedic treatment. Many patients with diseases that are not readily amenable to modern treatments have benefited greatly from the use of Ayurvedic therapeutic measures.

On the other hand, in Ayurveda there is no effective method for managing such acute emergencies as perforated peptic ulcer. Here the responsibility of the Ayurvedic physicians is to make a correct diagnosis promptly and refer the patient to a specialist for the necessary treatment. It is essential that Ayurvedic physicians are competent enough to differentiate these acute emergencies and to take prompt action.

Medicines for external application

In addition to the administration of internal medicines, Ayurveda prescribes a large number of medicines for external use in the form of pastes, medicated oils for massage, medicated baths, gargles, and powders. The efficacy of medicated oils for treating some diseases of the joints and also neuromuscular disorders is well known.

The treatment of burns with specific external applications is also well established. In cases of early superficial burns, ointments prepared from papaya juice are applied to produce gradual *débridement* of devitalized and dead tissues. When this process is completed and the healthy granulation tissues appear, the local application of medicated *ghee* prepared from the *jati* flower promotes healing. In extensive burns, such treatment is supplemented by skin grafting to replace lost tissue.

Surgical treatment

Ayurveda describes in great detail various surgical conditions and their management. These include different types of fracture and the principles of their management and various operative and palliative treatments for surgical conditions such as urinary stones, piles, fistulae, goitre, lymphadenitis, hernia, and hydrocele. Many plastic operations such as rhinoplasty and auroplasty have been described in detail; likewise the ambulatory treatment of fistula in ano with corrosive threads has been advised in preference to the extensive excision of fistulous tracks, which requires confinement to bed for several days and involves the risk of secondary infection.

Psychosomatic treatment

Although treatment has been described in detail for different diseases, the Ayurvedic physician is required to individualize therapy with regard to drug components and ingredients, dosage, diet, and rest, according to the psychosomatic constitution of the individual patient and also the predominance of vitiated humours in the disease process. In cases of psychiatric ailment, certain prayers and offerings are made to the gods in order to allay the harmful effects of evil spirits on the patients and their families.

The status of Ayurvedic practitioners

In India there are at present about 50 000 institutionally qualified practitioners and about 150 000 non-institutionally qualified registered practitioners of Indian medicine, including the Ayurvedic, Unani, and Sidha systems of medicine. In addition, it is estimated that there are another 200 000 traditional Ayurvedic practitioners practising in the rural areas who are neither qualified from any institute nor registered with any state council. These practitioners receive practical in-service training from their preceptors. Most of them use only Ayurvedic medicines prepared by themselves or purchased from Ayurvedic dispensaries. However, the institutionally qualified practitioners also employ modern drugs, mostly for acute conditions. Ayurvedic drugs are generally preferred by people living in rural communities. Most Ayurvedic physicians are local residents and remain very close to the people socially and culturally. They are also able to gain the full confidence of the community, and in spite of all the modern advance in medicine, Ayurvedic physicians remain very popular and highly respected, especially in rural India.

There is a wide divergence of standards of payment for the services rendered by these Ayurvedic physicians, varying from Rs 2 to Rs 10 ($0.25–1.2) per visit, depending upon the type of training the practitioner has had. Most of the traditionally trained Ayurvedic physicians have had their basic education in Sanskrit before undertaking Ayurveda. The pure Ayurvedic physicians undergo training in an institution for 4 years after matriculation whereas the integrated Ayurvedic graduates undergo 4½–5 years' training after the intermediate examination, just as modern medical (M.B., B.S.) graduates do.

About 10% of those qualified and registered as Ayurvedic physicians seek government service and work in rural Ayurvedic dispensaries. However, in most states their salary and status are much lower than those of modern medical graduates. Many Ayurvedic physicians therefore prefer to go into private practice in the rural areas.

The state and central governments support about 9000 Ayurvedic dispensaries and 195 hospitals that offer services to the people mainly according to the Indian system of medicine. They are usually manned by institutionally trained and qualified Ayurvedic physicians.

The role of Ayurveda in modern medicine

Review of the training curriculum

The Ayurvedic system of medicine has remained with the people as part of their culture for many generations. Traditionally trained Ayurvedic physicians used to meet the primary health needs of the people in the rural areas at a very low cost, since their medicines are cheaply prepared from the herbs readily available in the fields and local markets. Nearly 100 Ayurvedic colleges have been established in India and have so far trained some 50 000 institutionally qualified Ayurvedic physicians. Most of these people have not only a good basic knowledge of Ayurvedic medicine but also an adequate practical knowledge of modern medical sciences. If additional short-term refresher courses were provided for these practitioners, they could become eminently suited to meet the immediate needs of rural populations by providing primary medical and health care.

It is clear that the ultimate solution to the health problems of the developing nations is a fully integrated type of training that includes the essential principles of both the indigenous system of medicine and the principles of modern medical sciences, so that practitioners can serve the rural populations with efficiency and understanding and at relatively low cost.

Earlier attempts at integration

Integration of the Ayurvedic system of medicine with modern medical science was attempted as soon as the latter was introduced in India in the early part of the 19th century. Since then many arguments have been developed for and against integration, and many committees have been appointed by different states and the central government to review the matter. These committees, including the one appointed by the Government of India, which submitted its report in 1948, recommended the integration of Ayurveda and modern medicine as regards education, practice, and research, stating that this was not only possible but most desirable in order to provide efficient medical relief to the people living in the rural areas.

The integrated colleges of Indian medicine have already produced nearly 7000 graduates trained in both systems of medicine. They started practising in the rural, semiurban, and urban areas and became popular with the people since they could use both Ayurvedic and modern drugs. However, these integrated graduates have become a target for criticism for economic and social reasons, and lack of government recognition has created much frustration amongst them.

In view of this, several states have recently changed their policy and now use relatively pure Ayurvedic courses to train Ayurvedic physicians with only elementary instruction in the modern medical sciences. However, some states and many private organizations continue to provide integrated training.

More than 5000 primary health centres have been established in India with about 30 000 associated subcentres. Many of these centres and subcentres are not functioning efficiently because of the lack of trained medical men. The doctors trained in modern medical sciences do not wish to settle and work in the rural areas because of the lack of facilities and social amenities. The so-called pure Ayurvedic physicians are not suitable either because they lack adequate training in community health and modern medical sciences.

Proposals for integrating medical education and practice

Integrated medical education

There are in India at present 107 modern medical colleges admitting more than 13 000 medical students annually and 102 Ayurvedic and other indigenous medical colleges (91 Ayurvedic, 10 Unani, and 1 Sidha) admitting about 7000 students annually, thus making a total of 20 000 students a year. These different types of medical institution run on parallel lines with no definite commitment on their part to render service to the rural population. This shortcoming can be remedied only by starting a fully integrated medical course in all the existing institutions.

The Central Council of Indian Medicine is at present reviewing Ayurvedic education. The curriculum that has just been agreed contains mostly Ayurveda with a comparatively small content of modern medicine.

Postgraduate training

The following is a description of the integrated postgraduate medical education system developed at the Banaras Hindu University.

The College of Ayurveda was established at the University as early as 1927 and initiated a 5-year integrated training programme in Indian medicine and modern medicine and surgery leading to the award of the degree A.M.S., and later the A.B.M.S. (Ayurveda Bachelor of Medicine and Surgery). A training programme in all fields of medical science was developed, but in 1960 the undergraduate course in Ayurveda was discontinued on account of the state and central governments' refusal to recognize A.B.M.S. as equivalent to the medical degree of M.B., B.S. However, the importance of Indian medicine was fully appreciated and a 3-year postgraduate training course in Indian medicine was initiated in 1963 at the College of Medical Sciences of the Banaras Hindu University. Admission to this course is open to graduates in both Ayurvedic and modern medicine. In the first year after graduation in Ayurveda (A.B.M.S.) the doctor has to undergo training in applied aspects of modern medical subjects, while the graduate in modern medicine (M.B., B.S.) has to study the basic principles of Ayurveda. The next two years are devoted to studies and clinical and laboratory research in any one of the five Ayurvedic specialities. At the end of the 2-year period the candidate submits a thesis and is examined in two papers on the subject of specialization. In addition, one paper is based on classical Ayurvedic texts and another on an allied modern subject. Successful students are awarded the D.Ay.M.

This training programme affords students the opportunity to acquire knowledge in both Indian and modern medicine and enables them also to undertake original scientific investigations with analysis of research findings.

Since 1966 a course for the Ph.D. degree in Ayurveda has been developed with a view to promoting advanced research in Ayurvedic subjects.

The Indian Medicine Unit of the Institute of Medical Sciences comprises the following six departments:

1. Basic principles of Ayurveda

2. Dravyaguna (properties of medicinal substances, materia medica, pharmacology)

3. Kaya Chikitsa (general medicine, therapeutics)

4. Shalaya Shalkya (surgery)
5. Prasuti Tantra (obstetrics and gynaecology)
6. Medicinal chemistry.

The University also runs a regular course in modern medicine for the training of students for the M.B., B.S., M.D., and M.S. qualifications. Admission requirements are the same as for other medical colleges. The general opinion is that the M.B., B.S. course should also include the essential features of Ayurvedic medicine in order to equip practitioners more fully for health work in India.

Research

The need to conduct applied research is evident, and in this field the Institute has made several contributions on the therapeutic value of Ayurvedic drugs, by determining their mode of action, by isolating their active principles, and by assessing effective dosage and toxicity. An anabolic steroid has been isolated from *Cissus quadrangularis* and has been studied extensively to determine its role in fracture healing. A catabolic steroid has been isolated that is said to be highly effective in the prevention and treatment of hyperlipidaemia and its complications, including atherosclerosis and coronary thrombosis. The herbal substances *jati ghrit* and *kshar-sutra* have also been standardized for wound healing and for the treatment of fistula in ano by means of suitably impregnated sutures passed through the fistular tract. Other drugs that have been studied include *Picrorrhiza kurroa* for the treatment of liver diseases and *Allium sativum* for the control of hypercholesterolaemia and heart diseases, and *Semecarpus anacardium-Bhallatak* is used for worm infestations and arthritis, *tambool* for heart diseases, and *punarnava* for urinary diseases.

In addition there is also an urgent need for conducting research into the practice of Yoga, which has generated worldwide interest in recent years. As already stated, different Yoga practices help not only to maintain good positive bodily health but also to maintain good mental health, peace of mind, and happiness.

In order to determine the best method of providing health care to the rural people efficiently and at low cost, it will be necessary to establish a few pilot research schemes in different parts of the country. Such operational research will have to be designed realistically, using available local resources, including health manpower, and with the minimum of external input.

Improvement in the health care delivery system

As soon as a large number of graduates who have followed integrated studies of both modern and Ayurvedic medicine are being produced in all the medical teaching institutions, they can be encouraged to serve in the rural areas and to man the primary health centres and subcentres. These practitioners should be able to serve the rural areas much better than graduates trained exclusively in modern medicine or Ayurveda. Those who wish to establish private practice in the rural areas should be given encouragement in the form of loans and subsidiary monthly allowances.

Meanwhile, the training institutes can initiate short-term training programmes for any graduates who are willing to become involved in rural health care. Thus modern medical graduates would be trained in the main principles of Ayurvedic medicine and pure Ayurvedic graduates would be required to learn the essentials of modern medical subjects, and both would function with greater efficiency and confidence. Furthermore, if such opportunities were offered to practitioners in the rural areas, it is possible that the so-called "brain drain" of graduates of medicine might be considerably reduced.

Conclusions

Official recognition of indigenous systems by the governments of the countries in which the practice is established would no doubt help in improving the quality of practitioners and promoting knowledge of the system.

Surveys of indigenous medical practices indicate that there is an urgent need for additional training in order to improve efficiency and usefulness. The training programmes should be structured so as to meet the special needs of the different categories of indigenous medical practitioner, and priority should be given to orientation in community and public health practice.

Practitioners of modern medicine and undergraduate medical students also require some orientation in indigenous systems where relevant in order to improve their knowledge and bring about the necessary changes in attitude.

The studies outlined above are considered essential prerequisites for the integration of indigenous systems into government-sponsored health services.

In India, an estimated 400 000 indigenous practitioners are functioning, —mostly in the rural areas—and could probably be developed and utilized to provide full coverage.

The idea of developing mass services or total health coverage for rural communities now appears more realistic than once seemed possible.

FURTHER READING

Banerji, D. *Social and cultural foundations of health services systems of India*, New Delhi, Centre of Social Medicine and Community Health, J.N. University, 1974

Castiglioni, A. *A history of medicine*, New York, Knopf, 1947

Cheng, T. O. Medicine in modern China. *J. Amer. Geriat. Soc.*, **21**: 289 (1973)

Dwarakanath, C. *Introduction to Kaya Chikitsa*, Bombay, Popular Book Depot, 1959

Giri, D. T. Indigenous practitioners and the rural health services. *Indian J. med. Educ.*, **12**: 253 (1973)

India, Ministry of Health. *Report of the Committee on the Indigenous Systems of Medicine*, New Delhi, 1948, vol. 1

India, Ministry of Health. *Report of the Committee to Assess and Evaluate the Present Status of the Ayurvedic System of Medicine*, New Delhi, 1959

Major, R. H. *A history of medicine*, Oxford, Blackwell, 1954, vol. 1

Mehta, P. M. et al. *The Charaka Samhiti*, Jamnagar, Shri Gulabkunverba Ayurvedic Society, 1949

Patel, C. H. Yoga and biofeedback in the management of hypertension. *Lancet*, **2**: 1053 (1973)

Rao, K. N. Global trends in rural health services. *Indian J. med. Educ.*, **12**: 165 (1973)

Shiv Sharma. *The system of Ayurveda*, Bombay, Khemraj Shrikrishnadas, Shri Venkateshwar, 1929

Sigerist, H. E. *A history of medicine*, New York, Oxford University Press, 1961, vol. 2

Swami Vivekananda, Raja Yoga, or conquering the internal nature, Calcutta, Advaita Ashrama, 1970

Udupa, K. N. et al. Studies on physiological, endocrine and metabolic response to the practice of Yoga in young normal volunteers. *J. Res. ind. Med.*, **6**: 345 (1971)

Udupa, K. N. & Singh, R. H. The scientific basis of Yoga. *J. Amer. med. Ass.*, **220**: 1365 (1972)

Udupa, K. N. et al. Certain studies on psychological and biochemical responses to the practice of Hatha Yoga in young normal volunteers. *Indian J. med. Res.* **61**: 237 (1973)

Udupa, K. N. Bodily response to injury. *Quart. J. surg. Sci.*, suppl. 2. (1973)

Vahia, N. S. et al. A deconditioning therapy based upon concepts of patanjali. *Int. J. Soc. Psychiat.* **18**: 61 (1972)

Varma, O. P. Present pattern of rural health services in India. *Indian J. med. Educ.*, **12**: 162 (1973)

Zimmer, H. R. *Hindu medicine*, Baltimore, Johns Hopkins Press, 1948

A COMPREHENSIVE RURAL HEALTH PROJECT IN JAMKHED (INDIA)

MABELLE AROLE & RAJANIKANT AROLE [a]

Rural areas in India do not have adequate health care. Children under five suffer from malnutrition, fevers, diarrhoeas; pregnant women do not receive sufficient antenatal care or skilled help during delivery. Inadequate, unsafe drinking water gives rise to waterborne infections. Chronic illnesses such as tuberculosis and leprosy are prevalent in various areas. Unchecked population growth adds to these problems. There is disparity in the availability of health care in urban and rural areas. These considerations led us to serve in a rural area.

How the project was conceived

After graduating from a medical school my wife and I worked in a rural voluntary hospital in Maharashtra State during 1962–1966. This 70-bed hospital was the only facility available for the 100 000 people in the area. It offered traditional western curative medical care to those who found their way to its doorstep. After four years of service we recognized that 70% of illnesses were preventable and large numbers of patients "cured" in the hospital were going back to the same environment and later returning to the hospital for the same sort of episode of illness. This repetitive pattern of simple preventable illnesses could not be changed by the hospital even though it was situated in the heart of the rural area. Since a traditional curative-oriented hospital system does not penetrate the communities and does not see patients as a part of a community in relation to the environment they live in, it fails to meet the total needs of the community.

Recognition of this fact led us to look for a system that would cover the entire rural population in a given area and meet the basic minimum health needs of the community. Working within such a system we could also show other health organizations how to meet the total health needs of rural communities.

---

[a] In collaboration with V. Djukanović, Division of Strengthening of Health Services, World Health Organization, Geneva, Switzerland.

Since we were isolated in a rural area and since we had to be competent to deal with various clinical conditions in the villages we both decided to undertake three years of clinical experience in medicine and surgery. To practise community medicine in rural areas we each took one year's training in public health abroad.

At the Johns Hopkins School of Public Health detailed plans for providing medical care for rural populations were drawn up. We had the opportunity of receiving guidance and criticism from others engaged in health care delivery in various parts of the developing world. Then, having finished our planned training, we returned to Maharashtra to provide health care for a needy rural area.

We had formulated the following criteria for establishing a viable and effective health care system. (1) Local communities should be motivated and involved in decision-making and must participate in the health programme so that ultimately they "own" the programme in their respective communities and villages. (2) The programme should be planned at the grass roots and develop a referral system to suit the local conditions. (3) Local resources such as buildings, manpower, and agriculture should be used to solve local health problems. (4) The community needs total health care and not fragmented care; promotional, preventive, and curative care need to be completely integrated, without undue emphasis on one particular aspect.

How the project was started

Before putting the plan into action we needed money to support ourselves and the other medical staff until we became self-supporting. We needed capital to put up buildings and buy vehicles and equipment. The Christian Medical Commission, through various religious and secular agencies, found money to initiate the project.

We decided to select a needy area in Maharashtra with a population of 40 000, which we estimated was manageable. Various communities in three needy and relatively underdeveloped districts of south-east Maharashtra were approached. It was explained to the community leaders that we were interested in meeting the basic health needs of the people through curative, preventive, and promotional methods, provided they participated actively in making a building available for health activities in each village, participated in active health promotional and preventive activities such as the mass immunization of children, and provided volunteers to help the health personnel in their work.

Most community leaders enthusiastically invited us to work in their areas. When we actually visited the communities, our experience varied. In one community the leader wanted to sell his property at high cost to "foreign returned wealthy" doctors. In another community, a local practitioner of indigenous medicine successfully prevented any dialogue between us and the people. Some communities felt that we were going to them because we had no practice in cities; most felt that we were merely outside professionals trying to make money in their areas; some thought that we had other ulterior motives.

Government officials in the area involved in health care and general administration were also approached and our plans were explained to them. They appreciated our decision to work for the rural people and promised support as they were concerned about inadequate health care in rural areas.

The project area [a]

Jamkhed is situated 400 km south-east of Bombay in Ahmednagar District of Maharashtra state. It is connected to the district headquarters town Ahmednagar by an all-weather road. A typical village in the Jamkhed area consists of a cluster of houses built close together. Different caste groups live in different sections of the village. There is free communication between different castes but intermarriages almost never occur.

Agriculture is the main source of livelihood, occupying 88% of the workers; 66% cultivate their own lands and 22% are farm labourers. Only 4% are engaged in household activities. Agriculture is almost entirely dependent on the seasonal rainfall, which is unpredictable. The annual rainfall is 508–635 mm; the rainy season lasts from June until September. Few farmers have wells for seasonal irrigation, which irrigates 8% of the land. On 88% of the land food grains—including cereals (mainly millets), pulses, and oilseeds—are produced; only 1% of the land is used for cash crops such as sugar cane and cotton. Usually farmers are very busy during the sowing and harvesting seasons, which last for 4–6 weeks each. There are intermittent periods of intense agricultural activity and periods of relative slackness.

Almost every village has a primary school and some larger villages have a secondary school. There are no colleges of higher education in the area. According to the 1961 census, 34% of the males and 10% of the females were considered literate. Ordinarily, village girls attend school for no more than 5–6 years. Only in Jamkhed and some larger villages do some girls complete high school. Parents usually get their daughters married soon after they reach the menarche.

A village celebrates festivals at all times of the year. Many events in a person's life are related to these festivals. These are the times when

---

[a] Source: Maharashtra Census Office. *Census of India, 1961: district census handbook, Ahmednagar,* Bombay, 1965. Jamkhed is a relatively less developed area in Maharashtra. It is not necessarily representative of a vast country such as India.

72

married daughters come to their parents' homes. Usually a women goes to her parents' home for delivery, especially the first one.

A group of 5–6 villages has a weekly market in a central village. Each village has a village council and a head of the council elected by the people for day-to-day administration.

The original health situation

In 1961 the population of Jamkhed was 73 153 (by 1971 it had risen to 86 592); 42.29% of the population were young (aged 0–14 years), 52.50% were aged 15–59 years, and the rest (5.21%) over 60 years. The population of the whole district has been steadily growing by 25% per decade between 1951 and 1971. The population density is 217 per square mile (84 per km ^{2}).

As for many other community development blocks, there is a primary health centre for Kharda block, into which Jamkhed falls. This centre in Kharda is 14 miles (23 km) from Jamkhed and has 2 physicians, 10 auxiliary nurse midwives, and 8 basic health workers. Including drivers, aides, clerks, etc., approximately 35–40 people work for the primary health centre, which serves a population of nearly 86 000. Each auxiliary nurse midwife located in peripheral villages of the block takes care of 10 000 people.

There is also a leprosy control unit covering 4 community development blocks, manned by a physician and leprosy technicians, detecting and treating leprosy patients in isolation and not integrated with the general health services.

The comprehensive rural health project at Jamkhed covers part of this community development block and serves 40 000 people in 30 villages. The project's administrative centre is situated in Jamkhed village. Formerly, health care was provided by an Ayurvedic physician heading a dispensary in Jamkhed village with 6 beds for normal deliveries. Another private practitioner trained in modern medicine residing at Jamkhed provided care. In addition, there were 4 Ayurvedic practitioners conversant with modern medicine, and 4 practitioners without formal training practised in 4–5 large villages. All the practitioners were male and practised curative medicine on a fee-for-service basis. Four government auxiliary nurse midwives were located in peripheral villages. A small drug store in Jamkhed sold Ayurvedic drugs. Patients needing diagnostic investigations, emergency care, or hospitalization had to be referred to a hospital 47 miles (75 km) away at district headquarters.

All the 30 villages are accessible by dirt road from Jamkhed. During the rainy season 7–8 villages are inaccessible for short periods. Public transport (bus) is available for 8 villages all the year round. The remaining villages have public transport during 6 months of the year. There are no trains or boats. Where a bus service is available it is usually during the daytime and 1–3 buses a day ply between the villages and Jamkhed. The main vehicle of transport is the ox cart; hiring an ox cart is much more expensive than a public bus (the rental for a day is equivalent to 3 days' wages for a farm labourer). Because of slow and expensive transport and the associated loss of wages of an attendant, most patients are reluctant to travel to see a healer unless the illness is serious or there is an emergency.

Study of outpatient data and surveys confirmed the national picture. Thus, malnutrition, episodes of diarrhoea, and fever among children were common. Baseline data indicated an infant mortality ranging from 80 per 1000 live births for Jamkhed to 150 per 1000 in a more remote community, averaging 110 per 1000 for the area as a whole. Most children had received smallpox vaccination but except for a handful of children in Jamkhed no one had received triple antigen or poliomyelitis vaccination. (In 1972 a district tuberculosis team gave BCG to the children in the area.) Most mothers did not receive adequate professional care during pregnancy and childbirth.

A family planning method (vasectomy) was accepted by 5–10% of couples of childbearing age in various villages. Oral contraceptives were not used and there was no facility for tubectomy. A few women had been sterilized in a district hospital.

The methods adopted

The community leaders were enlightened and influential. Some of them knew us. These leaders understood our plans and invited us to work in the area. They took us around to the various villages and introduced us and the programme to the communities. They helped to remove suspicions and doubts from the minds of the villagers.

Jamkhed is the central village of the area with a weekly market, government offices, banks, a high school, and bus connexions with various villages —i.e., a good centre for a catchment area. We had a series of meetings with the community leaders and explained our programmes to them. I doubt whether many really understood our programme at that time. Most of them were very happy to welcome us and to have curative facilities so close to them. We persisted in explaining our total health programmes and the need for participation. An advisory committee was formed. Care was taken to include local leaders representing various castes and various political party members. Their function is to guide us in health care programmes and provide a liaison between the villages and the project. They help us to decide how to meet community needs and to formulate broad policies. A small working group meets once every 3–4 months and a large group meets once or twice a year.

In our initial encounter with the community we made it quite clear that we should test them for the first six months and if there was compatibility we should think of settling there.   In the meantime we had recruited nurses, auxiliary nurse midwives, and paramedical workers totalling about 20 people.   Jamkhed community, with its limited resources, lack of running water, and lack of good housing, converted a storage house 60 feet by 30 feet (18 m by 9 m) into a house for 20 people.   The old veterinary dispensary was patched up to make a simple clinic.   Ordinary public and private houses were converted into an X-ray room, laboratory, and a simple "operating room".   Patients needing emergency surgery and close supervision were also housed in these facilities provided by the community. The community did its best to provide us with accommodation.   As work progressed a local farmer donated 7 acres (2.8 ha) of land on which to put up permanent buildings.   The community provided volunteers to plan and supervise the building work.   Similarly, communities from surrounding villages invited us to extend our services to them and offered help in the form of facilities and volunteers to assist health personnel. Some communities repaired access roads so that the health team could reach them. Youth groups also assisted in the programmes.   One group in Jamkhed has been donating blood for emergencies.

In October 1970, with the blessing of the community leaders and government officials, we began our work in the makeshift clinic.   For the first 3–4 months we were kept very busy by patients who had for some time been going elsewhere for the treatment of their chronic ailments.   Also, there were typical problems such as malnutrition, fevers, and diarrhoeas. There were surgical and obstetric emergencies.   Initially 200–250 patients visited the clinic daily, but gradually, after the backlog of chronic patients had been dealt with, we had a manageable number of patients.   The patients always paid a reasonable amount for treatment, indigents getting free service.   But this was not what we wanted to do; we wanted to give total health care to everyone in the area.

Our interest lay mainly in the villages around and equal emphasis had to be given to prevention and health promotion.   Popularity and reputation gained in clinical service had to be used as a springboard for launching community health programmes.   Acquaintances made at the centre were useful as points of entry to the villages.   A child cured of whooping-cough or tetanus was used as a demonstration case for health teaching in his own village and the community was motivated to organize a mass immunization programme.

Food and water take priority over health.

When the project began the area was facing drought.   We would visit a village in the late evening and over a cup of tea just talk to the village council members and other leaders.   These intimate contacts soon made us realize that their priorities were not health but food and water.

We began with food. We focused the people's attention on the most vulnerable groups—under-fives and mothers. Since there was not enough food in the area it had to be acquired. We took on the responsibility for finding the source of food. People organized a community kitchen. They found firewood, large cooking vessels, and volunteers to cook food every morning and to keep records. Thus the felt need for food was translated into the development of a nutrition programme. We could not continue on borrowed food; local resources were necessary. The community organized the digging of wells in the fields. The farmers who benefited from the water then donated land to grow food for these programmes. During the drought some farmers lost their animals and land could not be cultivated. Community leaders suggested finding some farm machines such as tractors to replace the animals. Jointly we approached donors to get tractors. Now the tractors do the work of animals on some fields and the crop is shared by the owner and communities for community kitchens.

There was a shortage of water. The community and the local government were trying to make water available. With the cooperation of the local government we got geologists from a voluntary organization in the state to do a survey. Medical firms, Maharashtrians settled abroad, and other agencies helped us financially to put in deep tube-wells of average depth 180 feet (55 m), fitted with hand-pumps. In this way a felt need for water was translated into providing safe drinking-water, thus minimizing the incidence of waterborne diseases. Local volunteers are being trained to take care of the pumps.

Agencies interested in agriculture and water development have been contacted and have helped to deepen existing wells by blasting and to supply good seed and fertilizers for the nutrition programmes. The project has a small poultry farm and dairy to meet the nutritional needs of the patients in the centre.

Just as we tested the community's interest in solving its own health problems, it too wanted to test us. Community leaders one day said to us, "There is a village beyond the hills. No auxiliary nurse midwife will stay there. They have communication problems. Could you provide health care to that village?" We readily accepted the opportunity. We found that there was no motorable road to the village. We asked the local community to repair the road. They organized community labour and we were able to make regular visits to the village. The community was divided and previously the nurse's experience there had not been pleasant. We had a series of meetings with the people and explained that a nurse would stay there and that her stay and safety would be their responsibility. The community cooperated and our nurse stayed there for over a year. A local farmer has donated land for the nutrition programme, and one of our best village health workers comes from that village. Our involvement in this community meant many rough rides on the road and many a blown tyre on our rickety old jeep but in the end it became one of our best villages.

Staff recruitment and training

As the work was progressing we were busy recruiting and training staff; we were trying to identify and contact all indigenous practitioners and health workers in the area.

Two Ayurvedic physicians with a knowledge of modern medicine were recruited with the idea of providing wider-based care to the people. A B.Sc. nurse with training in public health was added to the existing staff of 4 trained nurses, 6 auxiliary nurse midwives, and 2 leprosy technicians. Two social workers trained in community development work were added to help coordinate various activities of the project. In addition there are drivers, clerks, and a few manual workers. In-service training was provided to improve the skills of each worker for his role in the project.

Each staff member knows that the main objective of the project is to meet the basic health needs of the population by providing basic essential services such as antenatal and postnatal care, deliveries, family planning activities, the care of preschool children and mothers through immunizations (smallpox, pertussis, diphtheria, tetanus, poliomyelitis, BCG), improved nutrition, the diagnosis and treatment of simple illnesses in the community, the control of chronic illnesses such as leprosy and tuberculosis, the provision of safe drinking-water, and hospital care for medical, surgical, and obstetric emergencies.

In order to reach the communities scattered in different villages and provide care it was necessary to involve the community, as mentioned above. In addition, it was necessary to involve all the health workers and indigenous practitioners in the area, to train and utilize staff in the most efficient manner, and, if necessary, to create a new cadre of health workers.

We contacted the indigenous practitioners, invited them to the centre, and explained our programmes to them. We explained that we wanted not to compete with them but to help them by providing simple drugs, enhancing their skills, and providing facilities for their patients. In return they were to help us with regard to nutrition programmes, immunizations, and the care of patients referred to them.

We also needed professionals to help us in the administration of the project. There is a Governing Body composed of the chairman, secretary, treasurer, and four additional members. The two physicians are *ex-officio* members. The constitution provides that the members of the Governing Body should represent various national voluntary health organizations, and one or two should represent the nursing profession. The function of the Governing Body is to review and approve the annual budget, appoint a project director, and approve the general policies of the project. The Governing Body has given the director full authority to appoint staff, fix salaries, and adopt rules and regulations for the functioning of the project.

The health team approach

For the effective use of manpower, the health workers should operate as a team rather than work in isolation. The health team consists of a physician, nurse supervisor, social worker, auxiliary nurse midwife, driver, paramedical worker, and village health worker. The members of the team are trained together and each member has his role in the delivery of health services. Most villagers identify themselves culturally with village health workers, drivers, and aides rather than with nurses or doctors. Therefore, the team members at the lower rung of the ladder are specially trained in health promotional work as they are much more readily accepted by the rural people.

There are two mobile health teams that reach various villages daily and return to the main centre. Each team leaves the main centre early morning around 06 h 30 in order to be with the villagers before they leave for the fields at 10 h 00. The team does intensive work (including house-to-house surveys and case-finding) in one village and follow-up in a second village. Thus two teams cover four villages and return to the centre after four hours of work. Travel time usually is one hour. After returning, the team members complete the records and help at the centre. One team covers two nearby villages in the evening between 17 h 00 and 20 h 00. The rest of the staff remains at the main centre. One afternoon a week there is in-service training for the health team. Evaluation of team work and difficulties are discussed at a weekly meeting.

The mobile health team is responsible for house-to-house surveys to identify and care for target populations, namely preschool children and mothers, couples requiring family planning activities, and leprosy and tuberculosis patients. The nurses treat certain simple illnesses in accordance with the standing orders and refer others to the physician for consultation. Patients needing further care are brought to the main centre. The nurse is the leader of the team. She supervises the members of the team and helps the village health worker in her work. The nurse supervises the nutrition programmes, follows up pregnant and lactating mothers, and follows up women using various family planning methods.

The paramedical workers make a field diagnosis of leprosy and tuberculosis by clinical and simple laboratory methods such as skin smear or sputum examination and follow up these patients. In addition, blood smears are taken from suspected cases for the diagnosis of malaria. The social workers keep in touch with the community, receive suggestions from the villagers, and communicate problems of the community to the centre. They coordinate project activities in one village.

The physician acts as a consultant to the nurses and paramedical workers. He gives field training to the staff and village health worker.

Each member of the team gives health education individually or as part of a team. Mass programmes such as immunizations and school health examinations are arranged periodically in the villages.

Traditionally, the sick villager is taken to a hospital for care. Because of lack of proper communications he has to resort to private transport which is very expensive. In addition, the relatives lose their daily wages. This economic hardship deters the villager from seeking prompt medical aid.

The mobile health team cuts down the transportation costs to the patient and motivates people to seek medical advice early, before the illness becomes serious. Simply trained medical workers can manage these illnesses with inexpensive drugs. In the absence of the mobile team, the main health centre would be dealing with seriously ill patients requiring skilled medical care, expensive diagnostic tools, and costly drugs. Our experience shows that the use of mobile teams of auxiliaries cuts down the cost of medical care. For example, if in one week 8 patients came from a particular village to Jamkhed for treatment of illness, the cost to them would be:[a] Rs 64 for transport (hire of a bullock cart at Rs 8 per day), a total of Rs 80 for drugs (the patients being on average slightly more sick and needing costlier drugs than if they had been seen at home), and Rs 32 in wages lost (Rs 2 per day per patient and per accompanying relative). If, on the other hand, the mobile team visited the village the cost of transport would be only Rs 20 and the cost of drugs would be only Rs 20–50 (since the patients would be seen earlier). Moreover, the mobile team would be able to treat other patients who would not have taken the trouble to go to hospital. The follow-up of chronic patients and health education could be carried out during the team's visit. Hence the use of the mobile team saves both institution costs and patients' costs.

In addition, the health benefit to the entire community through the promotional and preventive programmes is enormous. For instance, if a child with whooping-cough is brought to the auxiliary nurse, she immediately informs the village health worker and social worker, who contacts the community leaders and, with the help of films and audiovisual aids, convinces them of the need to immunize all the children with triple antigen. A mass programme is immediately arranged and, with cooperation from the community, over 80% of the children are immunized.

The village health worker

Originally we thought of placing an auxiliary nurse midwife in each village to provide continuous care. It was difficult to persuade these young unmarried women to stay in a village; they were afraid to stay alone. So we selected some young unmarried men from among our staff of para-

---

[a] Rs 7.50 = US $1.00 (1974).

medical workers and clerks. As a result of match-making on our part, three auxiliary nurse midwives married young men on the staff. They still did not want to go and stay in the village. "We are going to have a baby now; how can we stay in the village?", they said. With difficulty a couple of them were persuaded to live and work in the villages. We soon realized that the level of their performance was not high although their salaries were substantial. We wondered whether the villagers could support these women in return for the service they rendered. We were doubtful. So we started looking for a volunteer from within the community.

The problems responsible for ill-health in rural areas are not complex and do not need highly specialized and scientifically trained people for their solution. These problems result from a lack of health education, an unhealthy environment, ways of living, scarcity of resources, and the community's culture. Undoubtedly, modern medical technology is necessary to solve some of the problems. However, to a large extent the community has to find the solutions. People selected by the community can be used to impart health education, change the community's attitude to health, and give simple medical care.

A village health worker is a necessary component of a health care system and not merely a stop-gap arrangement. City-trained health workers talk differently, dress differently, and have a different way of life from the village folk. This produces barriers between the health worker and the villagers and results in poor communication between the villager and the worker.

On the other hand, a person chosen from the community and trained is accepted and health promotion can be easily achieved through her. The village health worker feels important because of the new role she plays in the village. Having once convinced herself of the various health needs she is able to bring about change much faster than a professional. The volunteer, being part of the community, does not need a separate house, protection, or special allowances. Since her incentive is not money but job satisfaction her services are not expensive and are within the reach of the community.

A large part of the work is concerned with women—population control, maternal and child health. The village health workers are therefore selected from middle-aged women who are interested in being of service to the community. The village council recommends three or four women and a suitable woman is selected from among them. These women are active, well-motivated, respected members of the community. They are mostly illiterate, and do not have household responsibilities.

In-service training is provided for the village health worker (VHW). She spends two days a week at the main health centre. Here she receives formal training in the health priorities of the project. All training is done with the help of flash cards, flannelgraphs, and other audiovisual aids.

She is given training in the use of audiovisual aids. The training is in the form of group discussions, demonstrations, and formal lectures.

Each worker brings vital statistics for the week. Deaths are analysed from the clinical history and valuable suggestions are made relating to the illnesses noted during the week. Clinical cases in the health centre are used for demonstrations.

Training is continued in the field by the mobile health team when it visits her village once in a week. Thus the village health worker undergoes training for nearly two days at the main centre and one day in her village every week.

A VHW begins her day by organizing a feeding and nutrition education programme in the village. Here, she pays special attention to underweight and malnourished children. She helps the mother to cook and to feed the child and gives group health education, using audiovisual aids. Children are screened for simple ailments such as sore eyes, skin infections, diarrhoeas, and fevers and simple medical care is given. Children are weighed and immunization schedules arranged in consultation with the mobile health team.

Pregnant mothers are seen and appropriate advice and simple iron and vitamin pills are given. Immunization against tetanus is arranged with the nurse. Most pregnant mothers are seen at least once in two weeks and any danger signs are reported to the mobile health team or to the main centre. The relatives, who usually conduct the delivery, are instructed in simple principles of hygiene and preventive measures. The VHW keeps razor blades and sterile thread and bandage for the care of the umbilical cord.

In house-to-house visiting the VHW identifies women of childbearing age. She distributes oral contraceptives and condoms. Similarly, women are motivated to undergo sterilization. In addition to motivating the patient, the VHW has to convince the mother-in-law, as she exerts great influence over the daughter-in-law. It is not uncommon for a well-motivated young woman to come secretly to the VHW for family planning advice as her mother-in-law does not approve of it.

The VHW collects vital statistics (births and deaths) in the village for each week. She must record everything she does in the village. Her son or a relative helps her to complete the records. Chronically ill patients with leprosy and tuberculosis are followed up and suspected cases presented to the mobile health team for confirmation.

Health education is the VHW's most important function. She not only receives training in the use of audiovisual aids but also helps to prepare these materials (stories, dialogues for puppet shows) and suggests ideas for producing audiovisual aids suited to local customs and conditions.

Each VHW has a kit containing oral contraceptives, condoms, simple drugs, dressing material, eye ointments, etc. Every week she takes a bus or walks 6–7 miles (10–13 km) to the main centre to receive her training.

A health promotion stall is constructed and it is taken to various market places and fairs, where the VHW arranges puppet shows, etc., and mobilizes the masses for health education.

A VHW usually works for 3–4 hours in the morning and a couple of hours in the evening that are convenient to her. Thus, she has enough time to carry on her normal duties. Each village health worker receives an honorarium of Rs 30.00 per month. Training, food, and transport cost Rs 50.00 per month per worker. (Rs 1.00 buys a cup of tea at the airport or is a porter's charge for carrying a package.)

The health centre

To support services in the villages, a main health centre has been established at Jamkhed. It has an outpatient clinic and diagnostic facilities such as X-ray, ECG, and a simple clinical laboratory. There is an operating room for emergency surgery and sterilization operations. There are in-patient facilities for 30 patients, 8 beds being reserved for deliveries and sterilization operations. Patients needing detailed investigations, expert medical care, or elective surgery are referred to a hospital in Ahmednagar. A close relationship has been established with this hospital and the senior staff understand the aims of the project and have visited Jamkhed. Periodically, an ophthalmologist and an anaesthetist from the hospital visit Jamkhed for special programmes.

In addition to the project population, a large number of people from the surrounding areas use the services of the main centre, mainly for curative care.

The project in action

In order to appreciate various programmes let us visit some villages around Jamkhed. The mobile health team reaches a village by 07 h 00. Community volunteers are busy preparing supplementary food for under-fives and mothers. They use an average of 50 g of cereals, 20 g of pulse, 10 g of coarse sugar, and 10 g of oil per child. Some children arrive at this place, set apart by the community, with their mothers or with older siblings. Today is the monthly weighing day. The health team and volunteers record weights; children not gaining weight are separated out for special care and instruction to mothers. The VHW normally supervises this programme; today she can discuss some special problems of the children with the health team.

There are pregnant mothers whom the VHW has been following up. She found new ones last week. They are brought to the nurse for immunization and for an initial check-up. The nurse also talks to the women who are regularly taking oral contraceptives and those who are about to start. These women and their children have received some personal care and the women now understand why family planning is important. They can therefore be given oral contraceptives or brought to the main centre for tubectomy. The nurse and auxiliary nurse midwife visit the mother who delivered during the previous week. The VHW helped the woman's relative to deliver her in a hygienic way and took care of the cord. The nurse contacts another mother who had tubectomy some time ago and enquires whether she has any problems.

The physician accompanying the team spends some time with the village leaders and sees patients needing special care. He finds time to use some situations to train the staff in the village. As the team leaves the village they may be taking a woman for tubectomy and a child with a broken arm to the main centre for further care.

In the afternoon let us go to a village that has a large number of leprosy and tuberculosis patients. Most were diagnosed by the paramedical workers from the clinical signs and a simple laboratory examination such as sputum examination or skin smear. All were confirmed by the physician. Some needed further investigation such as fluoroscopy or X-ray. These patients receive regular care on a weekly basis. Their contacts receive prophylactic drugs (dapsone for leprosy and INH for tuberculosis).

Leprosy patients are not detected or treated in isolation. They are treated together with other patients needing help. Both in the field and in the hospital, leprosy is integrated with general health care. The VHW and paramedical workers are specially instructed to detect the early signs of leprosy and tuberculosis and the VHW keeps in contact with the patients. If they tire of the treatment she persuades them to continue. She dresses the ulcers of leprosy patients. Patients with anaesthetic feet receive proper shoes to prevent further damage. Some chronically ill patients cannot work; a project has been supplying them with goats for breeding so that they can make a living.

While the mobile health team is working in the field, another physician and staff at the main centre are busy with referrals from the periphery. The morning inpatient rounds are made; there may be a couple of tubectomy operations to be performed. A child may be brought in with dehydration or there may be a mother needing a forceps delivery or a Caesarian operation. There are other patients needing curative care.

This is the way programmes are planned for under-five care, family planning, antenatal care, and the care of chronic diseases in the villages, with support services at the centre. These programmes are planned so that care is available to the community at all times. Curative care is available at all stages and health teams and physicians are equipped to deal with common emergencies.

To strengthen the programmes, staff members are constantly being trained. Tuesday afternoon is reserved for mobile team training; Friday noon to Saturday evening is reserved for the training of VHWs.

Each Wednesday evening, village leaders from two of the villages are invited for an informal meeting over a cup of tea. This gives an opportunity to reciprocate the hospitality extended to the health team in the villages. The leaders meet the staff and see the health centre, so that they have the opportunity to see village health problems from a different angle. Interpersonal relationships built up in this way give them a stronger sense of belonging to the programme.

Similarly, members of the advisory committee meet informally about once a month. Problems of mutual interest are discussed, solutions sought, and experiences and opinions exchanged. Suggestions are made for improving the existing programmes.

The progress made

It is nearly four years since two physicians, uncertain of the future and with a few brave companions largely unknown to the masses, entered the area to serve the people. A senior nurse recalls: "On our first journey to Jamkhed we all started out in two jeeps with baggage in the trailer one afternoon from Ahmednagar to Jamkhed. It was raining all the way. The old canvas top did not keep us from getting wet. Streams were flooded and the jeeps could not go through so we had to wait in three places until the waters receded. By the time we reached Jamkhed it was dark. The house we were supposed to live in had only three walls and the front closed by a few wooden boards. Rain water was all over the mud floor. The bedding was wet and the food gone cold. I had tears in my eyes and said to myself, 'Why did I leave a comfortable house and a good job to follow these crazy people?' " Now she is the pillar of the project.

The project has penetrated all 30 villages and reached the target population of the area. Adequate staff are recruited, trained, and reoriented for the job in hand. One nurse with typical hospital orientation threatened to resign if she was sent out of the hospital to any village. This nurse's attitude has changed completely and she is now our best team leader, visiting rural communities daily. A physician had once to tell a group of hospital-oriented nurses, "I can teach a chimpanzee how to give an injection but I need human beings to go to the villages and change the attitudes of the masses towards health." Twenty villages have VHWs and more and more volunteers are coming forward to serve the remaining villages. VHWs have convinced the villagers of their worth and communities are being approached to support them. Community kitchens are becoming popular and, there are at present 20 villages caring for 2500 children. In one village, because of internal wrangling, the community kitchen was closed down. After 8 months the villagers noticed that their children were losing weight and restarted the nutrition programme. Mothers who objected to immunization are now willingly bringing their children and paying for this service. Most under-fives are immunized with triple antigen and poliomyelitis vaccine. Villagers notice that their children are gaining weight. This has led individual farmers to make 350 acres of land available for nutritional programmes. All 30 villages get safe drinking-water from 40 deep tube-wells. In the field of family planning, women now think in terms of spacing; 522 women are regularly using oral contraceptives. During this period 748 women and 301 men have undergone sterilization operations. The VHWs have convinced the mothers to accept antenatal care; over 50% of the pregnant mothers in the area receive this care regularly.

The project has been able to integrate leprosy care completely with general health services. General patients share a bench with leprosy patients in outpatient clinics; no one objects when a leprosy patient is admitted for treatment in a general ward. Early cases are detected and given regular treatment. Over 60% of the 353 leprosy patients are actively working. Similarly, all the patients with tuberculosis are on domiciliary treatment.

Results of the project in a typical village

This is what happens in a small village with a population of 1700 with this kind of programme. The people live in the same houses as before and do the same agricultural work as before, and their income has not changed much. But now they do not go to streams or rivers for water; they draw clean water from the pump. There is not sufficient milk in the village but mothers are no longer afraid to give solid food even to eight-month-old babies; this was unheard of before. Pulses and peanuts were considered bad for the child. A mother no longer stops feeding her baby because it has a fever. She now gives plenty of water to a child with diarrhoea. Formerly, women would not give fluids to a baby with diarrhoea, the argument being that if water is withheld diarrhoea or vomiting will stop. When a child is sick he now gets simple care immediately.

Last year most children were immunized against diphtheria, whooping-cough, tetanus, and polio. There are no longer epidemics of whooping-cough. The main health centre does not see nearly so many dehydrated babies and cases of severe malnutrition as before. Measles is frequent, particularly during the summer; no vaccine is available yet. But the mothers no longer hide the child in the hut saying, "Only Goddess can save the child". They take medicines to relieve pain, fever, and the complications of the illness.

Last year 15 women underwent tubectomy (so far 64 women have been sterilized). At present 40 women are taking oral contraceptives. Pregnant mothers are visited frequently by the village health worker. A nurse sees each of them at least four times during pregnancy and immunizes them against tetanus. Relatives of the mother still conduct most of the deliveries but the VHW is often present to help. There are still a few women who think they do not need care. "Where did I have any vitamins and injections before? I still had my babies. Why should I bother to take medicine?", they argue. But their number is dwindling fast. One mother blamed the tetanus injection when her baby was born with a cleft lip. These examples underline the need for continuous health education.

The health team and VHWs have identified 22 cases of leprosy and tuberculosis; these patients receive regular treatment, being seen once or twice a week.

Supplementary food is received by 200 under-fives and mothers every morning. Their average weight has gone up. The nearby fields look green with crops that will help the children to grow. The health team has been visiting the village every week. Sometimes it failed to appear, perhaps because heavy rain prevented it from crossing a stream, perhaps because the jeep broke down and lay in a garage for a week. They have cared for 720 patients in a year.

I cannot help recalling a shy, timid woman whom we saw a couple of years ago. Today she is the proud health worker of the community. It is a joy to see this woman with her head held high, carrying the health kit, walking on the main road of the village, visiting houses, joyfully imparting new knowledge she has received.

In order to provide this kind of service to the individual village, it costs Rs 150 per month for salaries and transportation, and Rs 2.25 per pregnant mother for iron, vitamins, and immunization against tetanus. Two doses of triple antigen and polio each cost Rs 1.00 per child. The cost of drugs for tuberculosis is Rs 7.00 per patient per month, for leprosy Rs 2.00. The average prescriptions of a nurse for 3 days cost Rs 1.50 and those of a VHW for a day cost Rs 0.25.

Financial aspects

The health programme is based on the needs of the community and the budget is in accordance with the programme. Curative care accounts for 30% of the budget, community health programmes for 60%, and administration for 10%.

Initially, capital investment for buildings, equipment, and staff housing was provided by donations from abroad. The communities' share was the donation of land, some building materials, and volunteers for supervision. Foreign donations for recurring expenses have gradually declined from 50% to 30% in the past three and a half years.

At the moment 66% of the running expenses are met from patient fees. The Government provides 4% of the budget, including cash payments for family planning activities and the cost of vaccines and drugs. The interest on capital received as donations from abroad contributed 15%, and a further 15% consists of donations from abroad.

It is expected that the Government will support programmes such as tuberculosis and leprosy control. (The comprehensive rural health project has had its own centre, buildings, etc., for only two and a half years; now that the position is stable, Government grants may be available.)

More support is expected to come from the community as it becomes more deeply involved in the project.

The present position

Where does the project stand now? The staff members have completely identified with the project; even when the senior physicians are away for a couple of weeks at a time their performance does not decline.

An attempt is being made to recruit and train a physician to direct the project. The project is now ready to train health personnel engaged in rural practice, to give them new skills to be more effective.

The project has made big strides towards being self-sufficient, a goal that it will achieve within a couple of years.

Some factors can be identified as being responsible for a positive change. Let us have a look at the physicians and the staff. Ordinarily, a health care provider sits in his surgery waiting for the needy ones to come to him. In the present project, the providers went to the consumers and, in addition, involved them in making a decision as to what they wanted. They took the risk of being misunderstood but, with the sincere motive of service, they succeeded in getting broadly based community support for the programme. Did special training of the physicians make a significant contribution? No. The training gave some useful skills and tools, but the success of the project is attributable to attitudes and personal qualities. Concern and compassion for the underprivileged, a willingness to identify with the masses, and the ability to withstand all kinds of inconveniences are the most significant factors.

Community involvement

Mobilizing the community at the grass roots, activating them to see their own needs, and involving them in decision-making gives the project a solid base in each community. Rural communities may be poor and less educated, but they are intelligent. They want to know "why" before they accept a programme. The explanation of health programmes through education accounts for the success of mass programmes such as immunization and the introduction of oral contraceptives.

Cooperation with the Government

A small voluntary organization working at the grass roots has made the concern of the Government for local health care its own concern. Its identification with the Government programmes is so complete that many villagers look upon it as a part of the Government programme. Yet there is no duplication. Joint promotional campaigns for family planning are carried out. Similarly, the project cooperates with the Government in extending services to the target population, providing immunizations and vitamin and iron pills to the vulnerable groups, identifying and treating malaria, and controlling leprosy and tuberculosis.

Coordinating the efforts of other agencies

The project has been able to identify agencies involved in general community development schemes such as agriculture and water development. Their services—improving agriculture by supplying good seed and fertilizer and developing water resources—are coordinated with those of the project.

The multisectoral approach

The multisectoral approach gave the project an opportunity to identify with the community, to make the community's priorities the project's concern. Health was viewed through the community's rather than the health professionals' eyes. This helped the project to be relevant and the project's participation in total community development elicited from the community a genuine response in favour of the health programme. Socio-economic development not only improves health standards but also enables a community to support health programmes. Agricultural development and water resources development are directly helping to achieve the health objectives.

The use of community volunteers

Originally the project planned to place several auxiliary nurse midwives in the villages to provide primary care. It was difficult to obtain them and those available were not effective. Local volunteers were used initially, as an experiment. Their value became apparent very soon. The use of village health workers made it possible to cover the population effectively and to give continuous primary care to people whom the health professionals had been unable to reach. The village health workers are an extension of the medical programme in the communities. In that sense they are an integral part of the project staff. Even if an auxiliary nurse midwife is available she cannot replace the VHWs, because their function in the existing village structure is unique.

The use of income from curative services to support community health programmes

For most people, curative care is a felt need; they are willing to buy it. Preventive and promotional medical care is not yet considered a need to the same extent. Curative care lessens pain and discomfort and gets the patient back to work within a reasonable time, but the results of community health care are not so obvious. At the same time, the delivery of community health care, needing transportation, staff, and materials, is expensive. In the absence of massive help from the Government or other agencies, the project is being pragmatic, using for community-oriented programmes the income derived from curative services.

The changing role of the physician

The physician alone cannot see every sick person in areas where the physician/population ratio is 1:11 000 or worse. He has to multiply his hands by training and using assistants. He needs to delegate responsibilities to others and supervise them. Thus, the role of the physician needs to change from the conventional one—an individual providing care for an individual—to that of captain of a health team.

The integration of indigenous practitioners

People need someone to go to when they are sick. Since modern medical graduates do not like to serve rural areas, indigenous practitioners often fulfil this important need. They are trusted by the community. This community trust can be utilized by implementing community health programmes through them.

Conclusions

Can such a project be replicated? The answer is "Yes". There are dedicated practitioners caring for people in the countryside. Communities trust and respect them as a result of their service. Each practitioner can be given responsibility for health care development in an area that he can manage. Governments and other providers of health care need to equip him with the necessary tools.

Similarly, medical institutions in rural areas can enhance their effectiveness by meeting the total health needs of the community rather than focusing their attention on the care of the individual patient.

The project is based on finding resources within the community and activating people to identify and help solve their health problems. Compassion for individual patients is an important component of medical practice. The same compassion needs to be extended to communities in areas not ordinarily covered by health professionals.

A COMMUNITY DEVELOPMENT APPROACH TO RAISING HEALTH STANDARDS IN CENTRAL JAVA, INDONESIA

GUNAWAN NUGROHO [a]

It was a sunny Sunday. A young couple knocked at my door. "Please doctor," said the husband, looking at the covered baby in the arms of his wife, "please, save my child". l took the cover off. A dying baby, stiff from the convulsions of tetanus neonatorum. "Please, doctor, I bring a rooster for you". I never did understand this, a rooster in exchange for the life of a baby.

And this was the beginning of an ideal—to love one's neighbour, to serve mankind. But it took a great deal of patience, perseverance, self-denial, and sacrifice before this ideal could be realized.

The background to the project

On the basis of experience accumulated over a period of 5 years in government service I became conscious of the need to review the current health care delivery system, particularly for the rural areas of Indonesia. The basic aim of providing primary health care had not been fully achieved and it became evident that the costs involved and the effort expended were out of proportion to the results obtained.

When I looked at the inadequacies, the lack of medical and paramedical staff and of health facilities, the immensity of the health problems, and the available budget (US$0.32 *per capita* annually), I knew that it was important to consider the possibility of devising a completely new way to raise the health standards of the people. The question remained, how far could this be realized, particularly with inadequate finance, staff, and implementation techniques.

Fortunately, in 1963 the government assigned my wife, also a physician, and me to the Foundation for Christian Hospitals in Solo, the second largest city in Central Java, with a population of approximately 400 000.

[a] In collaboration with A. el Bindari Hammad, Division of Strengthening of Health Services, World Health Organization, Geneva, Switzerland.

The foundation had existed since 1950, its aim being to coordinate church activities in the health field throughout Central Java. In the western outskirts of Solo, the foundation had a small maternity clinic of 20 beds with an outpatient clinic attached. Because of its location, a large number of the patients came from the edge of the town and the surrounding villages, the majority belonging to the economically depressed group. Daily management was in the hands of a midwife and auxiliary nurses, under the supervision of a doctor who came at certain appointed times. Occasionally financial support and equipment were received from private organizations overseas. This was the situation until the beginning of 1963.

The experiment

Drawing on my own and others' experience and attempting as close an adaptation to local conditions as possible, 1 tried to formulate some basic principles that could be used as a new foundation for drawing up a working programme.

It seemed to me that the maternity clinic mentioned above could be used as a base for providing health care activities for the surrounding areas. After studying the location of the clinic, its possible tasks and functions in the community, the staff and its capabilities, the general health services, the need for medical care in the area, and other problems related to health care and to resources that could be exploited, I formulated a simple and inexpensive working programme. My conclusion was that this programme should attempt more than merely serving those who came for treatment or those requiring treatment and more than merely preventing disease. The problem of health was not exclusively one of disease alone; health had a very close relationship with all aspects of life. A health programme should promote the concept of how to live a healthy life. At such an early stage this thinking was too far-sighted.

With no experience and no access to literature or experts who could assist me in the planning, I took an experimental road with common sense as the sole guide. The programme should be simple and inexpensive in that it should be in accordance with our own capabilities in terms of finance, staff, and equipment, adapted to local needs, and integrated into a wider programme, including the improvement of various other aspects of life.

I felt strongly that the provision of a health service should not always be dependent on overseas experts and aid; somehow a way must be discovered of progressing independently of outside assistance.

In order to achieve this aim, it was essential that the maternity clinic should be reorganized as a base and drastically "cleaned up" . This cleaning up was carried out first of all by improving conditions for the staff and increasing their wages to an adequate level. Discipline was enforced and those who were not prepared to change their attitude and to adapt themselves to the new situation either resigned or were dismissed.

In spite of considerable opposition and thanks to the resoluteness of the leadership, at the close of 1965 it could finally be said that these efforts had succeeded. The staff were now conscious of their respective duties, diligent, and responsible and, moreover, success had been achieved in cultivating the feeling that they also shared in the ownership of the clinic. The leadership was very conscious that the success of this type of broad health service very much depended on the enthusiasm of the staff in carrying out their respective duties. Good teamwork and team opinion had to be developed and carefully nurtured.

First the maternity clinic was upgraded to become a maternity hospital where abnormal cases could be assisted; it was also equipped with a children's ward and a family planning clinic. The idea was that the base hospital should also function as a referral hospital for the surrounding health facilities; it could also be run with greater financial efficiency as a maternity hospital. The improvement in the health care provided by the hospital was carried out by simplification in all fields. Deliberately, expensive and complicated equipment was not used; for example, in place of an incubator a glass box heated with an electric light was used, because most of the paramedical staff were young village girls with little education who were not capable of using and caring for the more complicated kind of equipment. Besides, it also had to be taken into account that in rural areas such modern equipment is not readily available. Through simplification, work efficiency was increased and there were considerable financial savings.

Auxiliaries were used because of the shortage of qualified nurses, but also because of financial considerations. It was also part of the family planning programme to postpone early marriages among unemployed girls by providing job opportunities for the girls, mostly drop-outs. Special courses were organized to prepare them for motherhood and responsible parenthood. Basic standards of cleanliness were observed and the patients' diet and the atmosphere of the hospital were adapted more to conditions in the patients' own homes. This pleasing atmosphere, together with an enhanced enthusiasm for work, guaranteed the continuing success of the improvements to the hospital.

The positive results from the cleaning up and reorganization were proof that the finance and work necessary to effect the improvements did not depend on outside assistance and this gave rise to a feeling of greater pride. This feeling of pride is working capital that cannot be assessed in terms of dollars and it increases courage and faith for further expansion. A sense of belonging and a sense of commitment began to develop in the staff.

From the information gathered in the outpatient clinic and observation of the surroundings of the hospital, the conclusion was drawn that the underprivileged group of the community was excluded from the health service provided by the hospital, mainly by virtue of the cost of the service rendered. An attempt was made to discuss this problem with the community through meetings organized by the hospital staff in cooperation with the headman of the hamlet and several prominent people of the community. But this gesture had been misinterpreted politically, so the first trial to introduce a "community health programme", in which the community would actively participate, failed.

The failure was taken as a challenge to find other ways of getting into the community. This was only possible if the doctor could spend more time outside the hospital. It was then decided that my wife would run the maternity hospital so that I could concentrate more on the community health problems.

Begajah

"A hot day, right in the middle of the dry season. A row of patients, mostly mothers with naked babies sucking the empty breast of their mothers, waiting patiently under the tree in front of the clinic. The nurse calling the names of the patients almost automatically and distributing milk and wheat. The serious cases were sent through to me and I was appalled as I examined the children, desperately looking at the patients' records. I shuddered at the thought that in another six months the cycle would return again, possibly worse".

Begajah is a village 20 km south of Solo with a population of approximately 3500. There were two outpatient clinics in the area; one government doctor was in charge of the government health service and I supervised the other one, while the daily work was done by a male nurse. This outpatient clinic was intended to be an extension of the maternity clinic in Solo. It was a poor area which at that time was always experiencing a shortage of food, with the result that each year many patients suffering from various forms of malnutrition came to the outpatient clinics. Appalled by the continual confrontation with malnutrition in its many forms, I developed a strong desire to get at the roots of the misery.

Activities began with a survey to collect baseline data but because of the political situation at the time further developments had to be postponed temporarily. In the meantime improvements were made to the existing outpatient clinic, which was converted to a health centre. This period was also used to get acquainted with the village infrastructure, the process of decision-making, and the socioeconomic and cultural background, through personal contact and observation. I found this the hardest time; having been trained to deal with the individual patient, I had enjoyed a privileged

94

position high on a pedestal, looking down at those who came for help. Fortunately I realized that unless I was accepted as one of them I could not understand the problems of the people I served, let alone help them to solve their problems. But how? Day after day, sometimes in the evenings, loitering in the village, having tea with the people in their homes, sitting under a tree and watching the women harvesting the ricefield, joking with the children, I learned a lot from what I saw and heard of the poverty and misery. I learned to speak the same language of poverty, to see through the people's eyes the life they lived, almost a routine of shortcomings and hunger, without any hope of improvement. I understood their apathy and surrender and, worst of all, their loss of human dignity. This process of change in my way of thinking and feeling took place slowly.

Having no preconceived idea or design, I drew up a flexible programme adapted to the baseline data collected from observation and personal contact. I was able to persuade the headman of the village and the local administration to set up a village development committee. This committee was responsible for the development of the village and it was agreed that the community should be involved in the process of decision-making through meetings where the community was free to express its opinion. The programme was thus developed from below with guidance from above. Development from below was the involvement, from the very beginning of the planning and programming, of the community that was being served in determining needs, decision-making, and taking responsibility for the activities. Providing guidance meant helping people to develop the will and the competence to manage their own affairs and, where necessary, helping in the technical implementation. This programme was flexible in that it was not tied to a rigid design schedule but was continuously being adapted to the changes in the local situation. This was the idea, but in practice the process developed at a snail's pace, which frustrated me many, many times.

Figures from the survey showed that the infant mortality rate was approximately 100 per 1000 live births and the nutritional status of the infants was on the borderline of malnutrition. It was quite obvious that the cause of malnutrition in this village was low food production. In 1966 the average family land holding was 0.2 ha of irrigated riceland and 0.1 ha of dry land, which could produce 480 kg of rice and 175 kg of other products such as soybean, peanut, cassava, sweet potatoes, and corn, if the weather was favourable. This was enough for a family to subsist upon, the average family size being 4.6 people. However, it should be understood that part of this production had to be sold for clothing and other needs. It was clear that heavy rains or a long drought would be disastrous for the village and this was the case in Begajah.

It was very obvious that the first step of the programme should be the improvement of the agricultural sector if I was to try to solve the problem of malnutrition, and for this purpose a community development team consisting of people from different disciplines and local community leaders was formed to assist the already existing village development committee.

Within this village development team the doctor could play an important role, if not a determining one, because in the eyes of the people his opinion as a doctor was beyond question. This was a very distinct advantage in a programme aimed at raising the people's health standards.

By using a demonstration plot, provided by the village, the team was able, in close cooperation with the government service, to introduce new rice strains, the use of fertilizers, and new agricultural methods. Through "food for work" programmes, in which labour was provided by the community in return for bulgur wheat, the irrigation system was significantly improved. For example, in 1969, through the "food for work" programme, 9.8 tons of bulgur wheat were given to the community in return for improving the irrigation canals and this produced an increase of 31% in the average yield. By early 1970 the rice production was almost doubled (from 442 tons in 1966 to 854 tons in 1970); this may be why, during the evaluation survey in 1970, when all the children below 5 years were examined, not a single case of malnutrition was encountered. During this period nothing particular had been done in the health care delivery except that health and nutrition education courses had been given to village women and girls. The infant mortality rate fell to 69 per 1000 live births. It was clear that this achievement would not have been possible without the activities in community development. Nutrition education in conjunction with increases in agricultural yields had accelerated the achievement of the goal. Viewed from the angle of cost and benefit, these activities were exceedingly cheap and yet produced effective results. For the first time, it had been proved that a comprehensive approach in raising health standards through community development, with community participation, could not only be implemented but was also cheap and appropriate.

I began to realize that the way in which the people lived had remained unchanged for many years. The gloomy bamboo houses without windows, musty and black with smoke, had remained the same. The model house that had been built as an example some years before was never thought to serve any useful purpose. The community had not been in the least interested, but now, after the standard of living had been raised and the community had reached the "take-off level", bamboo walls were gradually replaced by brick walls, windows were put in the houses, glass tiles were used, and the gardens were well kept. The smiles, the sound of music in the homes, the laughter of the children, the rippling paddyfields were all signs that the village had recovered from its misery. The community was proud of its achievement and had regained its dignity. It was on its way to a better life. We, the community development (CD) staff, the health centre staff, my wife and I shared in this pride and satisfaction. The team's morale was high. Looking over the green paddyfields, we wondered: what next ?

The development was financed by an initial donation of US$50 from overseas and the running costs and salary of the staff were covered by the base hospital in Solo.

After the period when we gained valuable working experience and formed a permanent team consisting of a doctor, agriculturalist, social workers, home economist, nutritionist, nurses, midwives, and auxiliaries (all paid from the income of the base hospital), thought was given to extending the project to other areas.

Sumberlawang

In 1965 the community of Sumberlawang, a small town with a population of about 5000, expressed the need for a health facility where the sick could be helped and treated. There was a government maternal and child health centre there with a midwife in charge. When I first visited the area I was struck by its poverty. It was a tremendous challenge for us to extend to this area the encouraging experience we had had in Begajah.

The sub-district of Sumberlawang, a barren area 30 km north of Solo, consisted of 13 villages covering an area of 80 km² with a population of 33 000. It was an extremely poor area, where food supplies were very inadequate because of the barrenness of the soil. To collect more information for the preparation of a working programme, I decided to open an outpatient clinic in one of the homes of the community. A nurse was in charge of this clinic and I came to see patients at least once a month and helped the nurse. But it was not until late 1969 that the work could start, because of financial circumstances and the absence overseas for a year of my wife and myself. Our absence from Indonesia gave us the opportunity to look at the programme objectively and from a different angle. The most important conclusion we drew was that the "trial and error" period was over and we should try to formulate a systematic method of developing a community programme that could be applied by others in different situations. It should be based on the most appropriate application of modern knowledge and past experience, adapted to local conditions.

While overseas, I was very lucky to have the chance to learn some techniques for doing surveys to collect baseline data and assess the health and nutritional status of communities.

Back in Indonesia by the end of 1969, refreshed and full of spirit, we returned to our work. My wife was once again in charge of the maternity hospital and the family planning clinic and I concentrated my efforts on the health care delivery around the hospital.

While we had been away, the outpatient clinic in Sumberlawang had moved to the new health centre building, which was completed early in 1970. The implementation of the Sumberlawang programme was carried out systematically.

The implementation of a community development programme is shown in the accompanying figure, which is, for clarification, divided into two sections: the technical implementation and the administration of the

IMPLEMENTATION OF A COMMUNITY HEALTH PROGRAMME THROUGH
COMMUNITY DEVELOPMENT IN SUMBERLAWANG

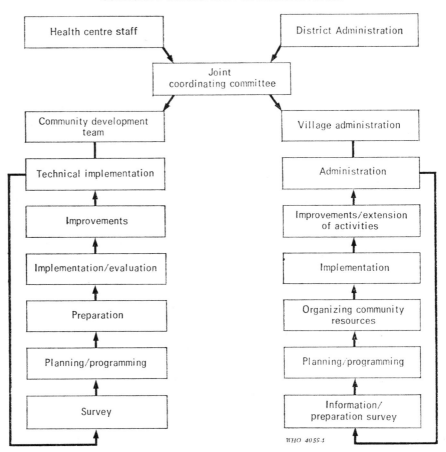

programme. In practice, the two aspects are integrated at the different steps shown, which start from the bottom up. The circular movement of the arrow indicates that the same steps should be taken if a new programme is introduced.

The barrenness of the soil in the Sumberlawang area made short-term improvements in agriculture impossible. The reasons for the poor health of the people could easily be understood. At certain times of the year they were lucky if they could eat a meal of cassava or corn and leaves once a day. The effects of this inadequate diet were very obvious when we examined the nutritional status of the people.

Survey results showed that of the 4000 children under the age of 5, 2.2% were suffering from severe protein-calorie malnutrition (PCM). The infant mortality rate varied from 100 to 150 per 1000 live births. The family size was less than 5, and spacing between the children was on average 2.5 years. It was clear that the basic problem was that of food production but improvements here were virtually impossible because of the poor quality of the soil owing to erosion. Moreover, the cultivation of the land on the unterraced hills increased the erosion.

The provisional conclusion was drawn that the urgent health problem was to save the 2.2% of children with severe PCM. The short-term need was an increase in food supplies and the long-term need was soil conservation. These "sub-subsistence" conditions could not be improved merely by providing health care, nutrition education, or environmental sanitation. Confronted by this situation, we had to make the extemely difficult decision as to what type of health care should be provided. A team consisting of local leaders and the CD staff was formed to supervise the distribution of milk and bulgur wheat to the families of the children with severe PCM.

This action had two effects, one of which was that it showed the people our good intentions. The initial reserved attitude of the community changed, aided by the presence of a doctor in an isolated community such as Boyolayar. "You are the first doctor who has come to this village since I was elected head of the village, some 50 years ago," said the old lurah (head of the village). The event was celebrated with tea and fried cassava, flavoured with joy and friendship.

Secondly, following our past experience, particularly that in Begajah, a local committee was formed, which was put in charge of the community development programme. Because improvement of the agriculture was only possible on a long term-basis, the CD team now focused on other available resources. There was enough grass in the forest and so the idea of goat and cow cooperatives was promoted but, owing to financial problems, the programme in its first stage was restricted to Boyolayar, the poorest of the 13 villages. Before it was implemented the programme was drawn up with the local committee, every aspect being thoroughly studied, to avoid failures.

Boyolayar is 43 km north-west of Solo and 13 km from the nearest main road. This distance over hilly, difficult country could be covered only on foot. The population was approximately 1600. Of the total area of 6.2 km², 0.2 km² (3%) was riceland. On average, each farmer produced 27 kg of rice, 3100 cobs of corn, and 100 kg of cassava annually. For an average family of 4 this annual production was sufficient to cover the food needs for only 4–5 months of the year. Water supply was minimal and depended on the rainfall. The nearest health facility was 13 km away. The infant mortality rate was 153 per 1000 live births. The nutritional status of many of the children under 5 was on the borderline of malnutrition, with a few cases of kwashiorkor. The average income per family annually was Rp 8000–10 000 (US$20-25).

I was completely lost, not knowing what to do and where to start. Looking around, I saw the houses of palm leaves with thatched roofs, and children clinging to their mothers, who were weaving bamboo mats. I went into several houses, gloomy and empty, the open kitchen containing the remnants of firewood and a dry jar; I wondered when the last meal had been prepared.

Paimin, a thin boy of 5, was sitting under a tree. He was licking at a piece of cooked cassava. In spite of being hungry after collecting wood in the forest he tried to enjoy his piece of cassava as long as possible. Joko and his sister with fever were alone in the house. It was about 11 in the morning. The parents had gone to the fields. There was no food in the house, or even water to drink.

Early in the morning the women of the village went out to the forest to collect teak leaves. With these packs of leaves, heavier than their own body weight, on their backs, the women went to the market, up and down the hills, a distance of 20 km, to sell the leaves for Rp 40–50, enough to buy 30 cobs of corn to support the family. How could these people survive?

Through the village ran a river, dried up in the dry season. Around the village in the brownish yellow hills, from which the top soil had been washed away, the farmers worked the soil in the hot sun, almost desperately, to grow cassava or corn, but unwittingly increasing the erosion. Suddenly I realized how irrelevant were my previous medical training, the postgraduate training overseas, and even the previous successful experience in Begajah. I was almost afraid to work in this area but the friendliness of the people despite their poverty appealed to me and almost forced me to stay on and try. I also sensed some tension among the CD staff. I could understand their reluctance to work and stay with the people, isolated, without radio, electricity, entertainment, water, or food. After a long and thorough thoughtful discussion in which I did my utmost to improve the team spirit and self-confidence, we unanimously decided to stay on.

The following days were full of action, spirits were high, and gradually we managed to acquire at least an overview of the situation, to know who was who, and to understand the social structure of the village. The CD team decided to start with a goat cooperative, since the possibility of improvement in agriculture was very limited. However, the grass between the trees in the 275 ha of nearby forest could be used to advantage for the goat breeding, which would increase the people's income and protein intake and provide training in cooperation. Local resources in the form of bamboo, straw, and labour were used for the construction of pens, the stress being on local participation and the expectation that people could improve their own lives. Nothing was given free. Fifty superior crossbreed goats were provided and one family would take care of two goats. The kids would be shared by the family and the cooperative. Every 6–8 months a new group of 20 families, selected by the village committee, was expected to take care of the goats. It was amazing how this simple activity increased the family's income by 30% annually, organized the community in a cooperative effort to improve the standard of living, and established a two-way communication between us and the community. The initial capital of approximately $750, to buy the first 50 goats, not only remained intact but was gradually added to and could be used for a new cooperative.

Most encouraging was the community's close cooperation. Together we built a school in the village. The previous buildings had been destroyed three times by high winds. More than 300 pupils, from this and neighbouring villages, had been meeting in private homes since then. Material was provided by the CD team through a donation from overseas, and labour and land were donated by the village community.

Health activities were mainly directed towards vulnerable groups—pregnant and lactating women and infants. The monthly weighing of infants was carried out during home visits by a midwife and social worker team using growth charts. Serious cases were referred to the doctor. As a result of this home visiting an outbreak of measles among 90 infants was limited to only 3 deaths. In terms of cost and effectiveness, this health care (home visits and weighing of infants) was extremely cheap. Data based on 2 years' practice showed that the average cost of care per child and mother was Rp 54 (US$0.14) per year, or Rp 272 (US$0.70) including the cost of the milk and bulgur that were distributed. The fall in the infant mortality rate from 153 to 43 per 1000 live births over a period of 2 years puzzled me. Was this because the health activities were geared to the vulnerable group?

A course for village women and girls was organized once a week, where they learned about health and nutrition, baby care, and sewing. The lessons in health and nutrition were completely adapted to local conditions.

In fact, in trying to adapt the health and nutrition education to the local conditions, I had gained more insight into how people could survive in extremely poor conditions and adapt themselves well to the environment. A week in this community taught me much more than a course in public health.

The home visits and the courses provided the CD team with invaluable feedback, which made it possible to adapt the CD programme to the needs of the community.

Young farmers were involved in the CD programme so that they could carry on the activities after the CD team left the village. They built fishponds in the rainy season, even for the short period of 4 months, to increase the protein intake, and a new grass strain was introduced to improve the quality of cattle food. Through "food for work" programmes village roads were built. This food distribution was also meant to prevent starvation during the critical months when there was a pressing food shortage. Given not as charity but in exchange for labour, it increased the self-confidence of the community.

The activities in Boyolayar had attracted the attention of the surrounding villages and requests for similar CD programmes were pouring in. It seemed that these villages were already conditioned to change and development. Armed with experience, confidence, and satisfaction from the Boyolayar programme, the CD team was able without too much difficulty to embark on an overall community development programme for the Sumberlawang area. Nevertheless, we often came up against difficulties in implementation, because it was impossible to know and to take into consideration all the factors involved. Experience had taught us that the process of change and development was a slow one with ups and downs, sometimes setbacks. Failures and setbacks, provided we knew the reason for them, were badly needed to prevent disasters occurring as a result of overconfidence and negligence.

By the end of 1972 our CD programme, of which the community health care was an integral part, had covered some 50 villages in Central Java with a total population of approximately 150 000. With the growing activity came new problems simultaneously from inside and outside. Foreign visitors came either out of curiosity or interest and this understandably aroused the suspicions of the local authority. Political tension has had its repercussions on this kind of activity. The coordination of the CD programmes in the different areas created a further problem. The pressing need for extra funds for the growing staff made me almost a beggar and hurt my feelings. The enormous mass of information and experience we had accumulated over the past years could be used for developing a comprehensive health programme, but it might all be wasted if we could not find solutions. I felt that I had reached the point of no return. But to make a decision was extremely difficult. I had the desperately lonely feeling of a single fighter, but a fighter for what and for whom?

A prepaid medical care scheme

I mentioned above that to serve the underprivileged group of the community in the surroundings of the maternity hospital in Solo a community health programme was introduced but failed completely because it was misinterpreted. Again, in 1967, with the advantage of some field experience gained during the previous years, I introduced the idea of a health fund. In the first stage this health fund, called *Dana Sakit*,[a] aimed at providing inexpensive treatment so that anyone who was sick could afford to seek medical care. The principle underlying the health fund was that of mutual cooperation, that is, the sick being supported by the healthy, a basic concept well known to the community in the past. Implementation was through a prepaid medical care scheme into which each member paid a monthly subscription. Perhaps because of severe economic pressures, or perhaps because of the failure of activities based on mutual cooperation in the past, or the fact that the people were bored with high-sounding proposals and empty promises, *Dana Sakit* received a negative response from the community despite the fact that considerable information had been provided.

In mid-1969, within the framework of a CD programme introduced by the maternity hospital, a campaign was conducted to clear the drains to prevent flooding. This activity was well received by the people because they understood its usefulness and also received bulgur wheat through "food for work" programmes in return for their labour. These CD activities were gradually made more concrete, so that a more extensive programme could be promoted. Within the context of this programme *Dana Sakit* was tried once again, this time under the name *Dana Sehat*.[b]

In order to gain a better understanding of conditions in the community a household survey was conducted, including enquiries into expenditure on food, herbal medicine, cigarettes, and medical care. Apparently the situation in this area was not too bad. The community was well organized. The average family income of Rp 5000 per month for approximately 5 persons provided them with at least 2 meals a day consisting of rice and vegetables. Health problems among the underprivileged were the result of poor sanitary conditions, housing problems, and ignorance of health standards. Information was systematically provided and discussions held, not merely on the scheme but also covering the wider topic of community development. It was during and through these meetings and discussions that both the maternity hospital staff, who would provide the health care, and the community, who would receive the health care, gained more insight into the health needs and demands of the community. It was understood that the minimum health care the people expected from the prepaid medical care scheme was the provision of inexpensive treatment for the sick and the introduction of measures so that the community could remain healthy. In other words, the objectives set for this experiment were:

(a) *Short-term :* 1. To provide a simple, practical, and inexpensive method of health care, adapted to the local situation and conditions and using the existing health facilities and available resources.

[a] Literally, "funds for the sick".
[b] Literally, "health funds".

103

2. To maintain adequate health standards in the community.

(*b*) *Long-term :* To raise the health standards of the community.

Of 17 RTs [a] in the environs of the hospital, RT 4 was chosen for the *Dana Sehat* pilot project on the following grounds:

— The leadership had authority and was progressive and far-sighted.
— The community of 301 people included labourers, traders, and also the less privileged, with educational levels ranging from illiteracy to university degrees; it could therefore be considered "representative" of the wider area.
— The RT was situated only 500 m from the hospital that was to be used for consultation and treatment.
— The people already trusted mutual cooperative activities following the success of the drain-clearing campaign.

The implementation of the scheme in RT 4 took place in stages carefully planned to ensure success after two successive failures.

Social preparation : (1) Extensive information was provided on the meaning, aims, and method of implementation, which was based on the following provisions.

(*a*) Each member would pay Rp 5 (US$0.0125) per month (0.5% of the average monthly income).

(*b*) Payment would be collected by a committee formed by the community of the RT.

(*c*) Each member had the right to be examined by the doctor in the hospital and to obtain medicines.

(*d*) Only outpatient treatment would be provided.

(2) Encouragement of the people to participate actively in the scheme and assume responsibility for it.

Stage 1 : A trial phase of 6 months, followed by evaluation. Depending on the result of this evaluation, steps aimed at improving and extending the scheme would be decided upon.

Stage 2 : Extension of activities to include preventive measures, health and nutrition education, family planning, etc., for maintaining the health standards of the community.

---

[a] RT = block. The city is divided into districts and the districts into hamlets. Each hamlet is subdivided into blocks, which have approximately 50–100 families.

Stage 3 : Extension of the scheme to other RTs and research into the possibility of providing a more extensive service, including hospital care.

The results achieved during the trial phase in RT 4 exceeded expectations. It was evident that the members understood and sympathized with the aims of the scheme. Stage 1 was then shortened from 6 to 4 months. Following this, RT 3, with 447 people, was selected as a further trial area and with thorough preparation (the same as for RT 4) the prepaid medical care scheme was begun. RT 3 was chosen primarily because there were pressing requests both from the chairman of the RT and the people themselves after they had seen the benefits of the scheme in RT 4.

It was clear that in RT 3 the scheme was also progressing well, despite a slight deficit, which had been covered by donations from the people themwelves. Only 4–5% of the population required treatment in each month. This proportion was much lower than the original estimate, which took into account the conditions in the RTs, the people's understanding and awareness of health matters, and also their economic situation. In this experiment nearly all the factors inhibiting a patient from seeking medical treatment were reduced to a minimum. The distance to the hospital was only 500 m, treatment costs were paid in advance in the form of a subscription, and the quality of the service was guaranteed, with a doctor providing treatment. Through home visits, untreated cases could be detected and the awareness and level of participation of the patient increased. From the financial point of view this trial was most satisfactory. The cost of approximately Rp 100 (US$0.25) per consultation, including both the cost of medicine and the doctor's fee, was covered by the contribution. A family of 5 members paid only Rp 25 (US$0.06) per month, or 0.5% of the average family income (compared with an average of Rp 85 and Rp 50 per month for herbal medicines and cigarettes). The scheme was able to provide the same facilities for the less privileged. The evaluation, using home visits and interviews, revealed that satisfaction was felt by the hospital staff as well as the people. All children under 5 in both RTs had a growth chart and home visits were conducted regularly. During these home visits information was given on matters relating to health and nutrition, family planning in general, and, if requested, personal problems. A two-way communication was established—a feedback system to keep pace with every change in the community. In this way, preventive measures concerned with specific environmental and socioeconomic conditions were carried out with the aim of maintaining adequate health standards in the community.

I was wondering why the scheme was progressing so smoothly and I was tempted to launch a campaign to extend the scheme to cover the rest of the RTs simultaneously, but fortunately I was cautious enough to extend it step by step from one RT to another. The next RT was RT 10, with a population of 514; after I had explained to the chairman of RT 10 about the social preparation and about how he could learn from RTs 3 and 4 the way in which it was implemented, I took it for granted that he would follow my advice.

Many difficulties were experienced during the implementation of the scheme in RT 10 but these difficulties provided much valuable information that was useful in the overall implementation of the scheme. The necessity for complete social preparation found justification in RT 10; prior to its introduction the scheme had never been fully discussed with the community, which had not been involved in the decision-making process. In fact, the dialogue that took place with the community through RT meetings or home visits provided valuable information on the attitudes and opinions of the people in relation to *Dana Sehat* and health matters generally. Members expressed a reluctance to use the scheme because they felt that there would be discrimination; for instance, they might be given cheap medicine or medicine that had passed its expiry date, or left to wait in queues. Others claimed that the attitude of the doctor was unfriendly and they therefore felt dissatisfied with the service. The rather inflexible attitude of the doctor obviously did not help to ease the misunderstandings that had arisen, but this could be partly explained by the fact that patients felt that treatment without an injection was incomplete even though failure to give an injection was justifiable on medical grounds and was in accordance with the regulations of the scheme. It was most interesting to note that the dissatisfaction was manipulated by the mobile *mantri*, [a] with whom the scheme provided serious competition. After several meetings and discussions with the community, confidence in the *Dana Sehat* was gradually restored and the participation of the community in RT 10 improved.

After a period of 10 months the scheme was reviewed to see to what extent it had fulfilled the hopes placed in it, in both medical and economic terms. The second evaluation, carried out 18 months after the scheme had been introduced, aimed to assess what difficulties had been encountered during implementation and the financial administration, acceptance, and benefits in relation to costs. The results indicated that more than 90% of the members of the scheme agreed to and accepted it and more than 80% stated that the scheme was useful and of benefit to the community.

Another interesting aspect of this experiment was the total cost of the health care provided through the scheme. In this total cost was included the salary of the staff providing the health care and the running costs of the hospital. The cost of preventive care—home visits carried out by a qualified midwife with extra training in family planning, nutrition,

---

[a] *Mantri:* an auxiliary nurse illegally practising medicine.

and child care, assisted by local women—was about Rp 70 (US$0.17) per person per year and the cost of medical care was Rp 60 (US$0.15) per person, a total of Rp 130 (US$0.32) for total health care *per capita* annually (excluding delivery and hospital care), an amount equivalent to that currently provided by the Indonesian Government for health care *per capita* annually. In this experiment the community paid a significant proportion (46%) of the total cost.

Over the years the scheme, which was introduced in January 1971, has grown and at present has approximately 5000 members. Most encouraging is the fact that the scheme not only functions but is progressing and developing on its own. To finance the community development activities that supported the health service, each RT had its own "central bank", where the members of the RT could invest or borrow money at interest. The monthly contributions to the scheme were also invested in this bank. The bank's profits were allocated for social and developmental activities decided by a special meeting of the members—e.g., to cover the deficit in the prepaid medical care scheme in the event of an outbreak of influenza or haemorrhagic fever, to build permanent drains and public latrines, or to cover stagnant water to improve sanitary conditions. Some progressive RTs were talking about housing cooperatives.

This was a community health programme within the framework of *Dana Sehat*, not merely delivering health care from hospitals to people's homes but effecting a change in the quality and the type of service so that it was truly adapted to the needs of the people. It had stimulated the community actively to promote and raise its own health standards without having continually to depend on outside assistance, relying primarily on its own efforts to solve its health problems. This community health programme had become concerned with helping communities to play a meaningful and creative role in making their lives healthier, i.e., more their own and free from the domination of not only disease but also other inhibiting factors.

The input or contribution from the community itself is a crucial factor determining the outcome of a community health programme as described above. Community awareness and a sense of responsibility, expressed in the involvement of the people in the community health programme, gives the programme an impetus that results in continuing and accelerating movement. In this way a community health programme that may require considerable input initially will in the long run become a progressively less expensive activity that can finally be borne completely by the community itself.

It is extremely difficult to describe the process of community participation, but it is certainly not difficult to learn the technique for initiating this process. One day the chairman of RT 14 came to me. "Doctor, our scheme is suffering a loss during the last two months. We have too many patients, twice as many as the other RTs. What can we do about it?" I was really very happy that this man came to me with this problem and not the other way around, so I suggested that a survey should be done before we could find a possible answer to the problem. A simple, quick survey was carried out covering primarily physical environment and health. The results, illustrated with maps, were presented at a meeting of the RT attended by the heads of all the families in the RT. It was as if the people looked into a mirror and suddenly became aware of the situation and saw the interrelating factors causing the increase in the number of patients. The clumps of bamboo, the stagnant water, the flooded latrines, and the crowded housing were all responsible—it was the community's responsibility, not the doctor's, not the RT chairman's. All agreed that rapid action would be taken to clean up the environment; this was started a week after the meeting and completed a month later. No dollars were involved, no experts, no outstanding leadership, not even dedication; what was needed was common sense, patience, honesty, and some imagination. Indeed, it seemed too good to be true.

Training

As mentioned above, by the end of 1972 the CD programmes covered some 50 villages (150 000 people) at a running cost of about Rp 500 000 (US$1250) per month. Although this was only Rp 3 (less than US$0.01) per person per month, this financial burden forced me to consider whether it was worth while to continue the programme, at least on the same scale. The community development programmes were not self-sufficient in the first few years because the process of development, particularly in the poor areas, was such a slow one. There has to be a substantial input before the community can reach a "take-off level".

Somehow a way had to be found in which this painfully acquired experience could be applied in other areas by other people. I decided to concentrate on the training of young doctors and nurses in the CD approach to health care delivery and also of those who were interested in CD work, in the hope that I could demonstrate that this approach was effective and reproducible.

Basically, the method of training was to develop the trainees' own ideas for solving the problems encountered in the field. It consisted of exposing them to the reality of the situation, to give them the freedom, through their interaction with the people, to find, cooperatively, solutions to existing problems and to mobilize existing resources for implementing a course of action. This meant that the structure of the programme evolved out of the problems encountered, which were dealt with in the order of their priority within the context of the situation. The trainess therefore knew that if they tried to impose a solution on the people they would meet with resistance arising from long-cherished beliefs; rather, they had to work out solutions with the people to ensure their cooperation.

The collection of basic data was then taught by the actual collection of information through participation and observation of community life. The trainees then met in groups (teams) to share and discuss their experiences, each problem being dealt with from various aspects. The solution was then agreed upon jointly by the trainees and the community. Some solutions were successful and others were not. The reasons for failure were further studied by the community and the trainees and different approaches were explored until the appropriate solution was found. Thus, the reality of the situation was used during the training as a selected framework for discovery, trial, and success. Involvement was the key-word.

The reproducibility of the programme

The following example provides an illustration of the way in which the programme can be replicated.

It was almost by chance that Dr Yahya came to Solo and talked about community health, while awaiting confirmation of his assignment. I was busy with the survey in Sumberlawang and asked him to join the team in the village of Boyolayar, which, for many of us, served as a medical school. When at last he was sent to Klampok, 200 km west of Solo, to start a health centre, he was determined that another, but better, Solo programme would be initiated. Well prepared, with the advantage that he could consult the team in Solo at any time and, if necessary, even ask the team to come and assist him in the field, he ensured that the programme was well off the ground in a short time.

After the health centre was built, with the help of a loan from overseas, he chose the village of Sirkandi, about 5 km from his centre, as the location of his pilot project. Sirkandi was a poor and backward village deriving its main income from palm sugar. The poor farmers had to climb the coconut trees to collect the juice from the buds in bamboo holders. The juice was boiled until it became thick, and then allowed to cool. Since money-lenders controlled the palm sugar business, the average farmer could earn only Rp 10 000–12 000 a year.

But Dr Yahya was able to perfect the CD approach in spite of the inevitable shortcomings and setbacks. Using the health centre as base, he developed a comprehensive community health programme, including a prepaid medical care scheme, relying on his cadre farmers to provide primary health care for the people. He had also developed home care for a variety of conditions, ranging from typhoid fever to accidents (falling from coconut trees), with results comparable with hospital care. The whole programme was based on health education, with active participation by the community.

The "mini-dam" built by the community with the help of a loan from the health centre for the material was finished in about 2 months and had a tremendous impact on the economy of the village. With an input of Rp 275 000 (US$700) it increased the rice production by an amount worth Rp 1 500 000 (US$3750) annually. Following the successful completion of this infrastructure, the community became aware of its own potential capacity, and activity accelerated to such an extent that malnutrition became a rarity.

In one village group, environmental sanitation activities were introduced within the context of the community health programme, initially by giving intensive information using a simple slide projector. All the activities were conducted by the head of the village group and the local cadre farmer, including the making of the filmstrip and its story. The role of the community health worker covered the training of the cadre farmer and the discussions with the head of the group and leading figures in the community. Lessons were also given on the making of filmstrips and a slide-projector was lent to the cadre farmer. It was most surprising that this villager with limited education could use audiovisual aids more effectively than we could. His own drawings and story were more easily understood by the villagers, who were semiliterate. Following the picture-show a most interesting discussion was held and just a few days later a spontaneous cleaning-up programme was held.

These and many similar examples showed that if a community health programme is handled well and the community is given the opportunity to play an active role, a programme that in the initial phases may require considerable input will in the long run become a progressively less expensive activity that can finally be borne completely by the community itself.

Conclusions

The general conclusion can be drawn that community life continues without any external intervention or any organized activities within the community itself. However, it is also indisputable that in order to raise living standards, concrete activities of an organized and planned nature —in other words, development—are essential.

A broad concept of development includes a network of activities, both physical and mental, to create the situation and conditions that enable a community to raise the quality and standards of its life. This network of development activities, which includes activities in the field of health, is in essence an application of modern knowledge to attain the situation and conditions referred to above.

A community health programme is one form of care that can possibly provide the ideal answer to the problem of raising community health standards in particular and the quality of life in general.

It is clear that, to achieve this aim, not only medical factors but all aspects of community life, including the interrelationship between man and his environment, need to be taken into consideration. It is even clearer that the application of this type of approach to health problems requires a radical approach. One must be prepared to leave conventional methods behind, not just because the idea is new but because it must be based on a search for the most appropriate application of modern knowledge and past experience.

A community health programme should include curative and preventive services and place greater emphasis on activities that increase the potential of man to live healthily. Educational activities aimed at the dissemination of lucid information about health and nutrition, the spread of disease and its consequences, the responsibility of a patient towards the general community and his own milieu, family health, and family planning are the basis of a community health programme. This information should be aimed at making the community aware of its situation and helping people to realize that they must overcome their problems themselves and not be dependent upon outside help.

The community health programme described above is certainly not a general answer to health problems or applicable in any place or country at any time, but is rather a framework; what should be placed in the framework depends on the local conditions of the community concerned.

There is no doubt that development activities that cover all aspects of life are not so easily implemented as expressed on paper. What is required is not a large amount of capital or a highly developed technology but leadership that is persevering, honest, not lacking in imagination and intuition, prepared to make sacrifices, and fully committed.

Many handicaps and constraints must be overcome but the most important are in connexion with people, whether they be the doctors, health workers, government leaders, or community leaders. The success or otherwise of a programme in raising people from the depths of poverty and suffering does not depend on outside activities but rather on the people themselves and their desire to awake and struggle out of the depths themselves. A community development programme is aimed at creating possibilities for the poor and the suffering to live a life worthy of man, with a reinstatement of their human dignity and pride. This dignity and pride cannot be purchased with dollars from outside; man has to create them himself by his own actions.

A HEALTH SERVICES DEVELOPMENT PROJECT IN IRAN

M. ASSAR & Z. JAKŠIĆ [a]

The project described here was first formulated in 1971 in connexion with a need, expressed at that time in Iran, to find a method of using national health survey data for health planning. A general objective was stated as follows: "To discover and test better ways to solve multiple health problems through an effective and efficient health delivery system".

At the beginning the approach was said to be "not to set prior task boundaries but limit activities by time and resources." The suggested approach included the following stages: situational analysis, proposals for alternative health delivery systems, implementation of a chosen system, and evaluation. The time-limit was agreed to be one year for the situational analysis, and two years for implementation and evaluation. One province with more than a million inhabitants was chosen as the field area for situational analysis and for the implementation of plans; this province was considered to be a large enough unit for the demonstration of organizational and managerial methods relevant to the whole country.

The background to the project

A story of rapid change

For the past decade, Iran has had one of the most rapidly rising gross national products in the world. The story of this growth can be traced through reports on the country's development plans. Because of this rapidity of growth, the country's plans were often revised. For example, the current Five Year Plan was expanded during the first year of its implementation (1973) as a result of the significant increase in oil revenues.

This economic growth has also been accompanied by many social changes. The programmes comprising the Iranian social intervention

[a] In collaboration with E. Kalimo and S. Litsios, Division of Strengthening of Health Services, World Health Organization, Geneva, Switzerland, and M. J. Anderson, Health Services Development Research Project, Iran. The work presented in part in this article comes from the Project. Dr A.H. Taba, Dr Ch. M. H. Mofidi, Dr K. W.Newell, Dr M. A. Faghih, Dr G. Soupikian, Dr F. Amini, Dr A. Khosrowshahi, Dr R. Manning, Dr A .Leiliabadi, Mr M. Subramamian, and Dr M.C. Thuriaux were very active in the design and conduct of the Project.

plan in 1962—called the "White Revolution"—affected many sectors and included the introduction of land reform, workers' profit-sharing schemes, an Education Corps, and a Health Corps, as well as a new status for women. In this manner changes were initiated that set the scene for a new social policy.

The short-term objectives of these programmes included evening out economic and social inequalities, raising the level of education, exposing tradition-bound rural communities to change, and improving housing and nutrition. These objectives were not only a humanitarian obligation and the declared right of the people but also a prerequisite for further development.

The health sector

A great many government, semi-government, and private enterprises participate in the delivery of health services in Iran. The total number of agencies and organizations involved is about 90, but 7 of them provide the majority of services. For example, there are approximately 45 000 hospital beds in the country, including the Red Lion and Sun Society's 13 000 general hospital beds and the Ministry of Health's 8 000 beds for chronic diseases. The remaining 58 % of beds are accounted for by universities and private and semi-private agencies. In 1972 the Ministry of Health directly operated approximately 400 health centres and clinics and—through an adjunct agency, the Health Corps (a rural semi-mobile service)—an additional 400 rural centres. Also in the rural areas, the Imperial Organization for Social Services (a semi-government agency) operated approximately 250 dispensaries. In addition, the Rural Insurance Organization—under the authority of the Ministry for Cooperatives and Rural Development—had a number of rural dispensaries; these were transferred to the Ministry of Health on 1 October 1974 as part of a policy of unification of rural health services. The private sector is responsible for approximately 18 % of the hospital beds and 7500 urban clinics.

The introduction of the Health Corps in 1964—a component of the "White Revolution"—must be considered as one of the more significant interventions. The Health Corps services nearly doubled the rural population having access to outpatient medical care. The Health Corps works as a semi-mobile unit concerned with medical care and the improvement of health standards in remote rural areas. The staff consists of medical-school and high-school graduates working as a team in fulfilment of their military service. Recently—under a similar programme—women have started serving as medical workers and health auxiliaries, extending the services of family planning and maternal and child health programmes.

In 1972, the Rural Insurance programme covered approximately 0.6 % of the rural population, the Workers' Insurance covered approximately 61 % of the workers, and the Government Employees' Insurance about

14% of the employees. All of these insurance schemes are growing rapidly, and their increasing role in development plans may promote coordination between the various agencies providing health services.

National health plans

The existence of so many health agencies makes it necessary both to coordinate technical activities and to encourage the most efficient use of resources, especially manpower. Previous attempts to resolve these problems are illustrated by the health sector objectives of the various national development plans. For example, the Third National Development Plan (1962–1968) defined health activities in the comprehensive sense for the first time; under this plan the Ministry of Health assumed responsibility for preventive activities as well as for overall supervision in the field of health.

The Fourth Plan, introduced in 1968, provided for the development of a new network of health centres to meet at least the minimum health needs of the whole population. The structure consisted of a major preventive health centre in each province, secondary preventive health centres in each district, and a comprehensive (combined curative and preventive) health centre for the rural areas. In pursuance of the objective of transferring responsibility for providing medical care to the private sector, loans were made to private institutions, insurance programmes were extended, and local community health councils were strengthened.

As the Fourth Plan was being implemented, the need to improve planning methodology became evident, particularly in connexion with obtaining information on the situation in the field for the purpose of formulating more realistic planning targets, and also with the definition of long-range prospects for the development of health services.

The Fifth Plan (1973) laid greater emphasis on the use of specific targets for attaining desired objectives relating to family planning, medical and preventive services, and nutrition (e.g., "It will be the responsibility of the Government to provide a minimum level of medical treatment services for the general public"). An additional and significant component of this Plan was the introduction of the system concept ("All units providing medical services will in some manner be brought within a single network of comprehensive and coordinated services...").

The origin of the project

Concern with planning

The frustration engendered by planning in the absence of adequate tools for implementation was evidence of the need to undertake health services development research. The initial steps in this direction were actuated by a desire to improve the planning mechanism alone, in the hope of achieving goals through a strengthening of the health services.

This desire was expressed in the form of small-scale experiments concerned with the operation of health services. Intersectoral research was also begun to assess the relative contribution of investments in health as compared with those in other sectors—education, communications, housing, etc.

On the basis of recommendations made by the Ministry of Health, the Institute of Public Health Research of the University of Teheran initiated a pilot health survey (the Rudsar study) as part of a national health survey consisting of six or more studies in ecologically different areas of Iran. The Rudsar study was an extensive project including the survey of a population of thousands and several intensive and special studies. The study yielded many interesting data on the cross-sectional morbidity pattern and vital statistics. However, frustration was caused by the inability to integrate these extensive data into a meaningful picture that could be of direct use for health planning. A new problem was evident at this juncture: health goals had been formulated, and the information on the existing situation was at hand, but there were no means of merging these two elements into an operational health services development programme.

Project formulation

In July 1971 a project document was formulated to deal with this problem. It defined the main goals, the expectations of participants, and the research strategy for the Project. A further refinement of concepts and delineation of study areas was accepted in February 1972: "to develop a methodology for health service development (of the preventive, promotive, and curative kind) in which the approaches to disparate health problems were harmonized for effectiveness and efficiency". The following five stages were described:

1. Specification of Project objectives and design (July 1971–July 1972)—with the participation of experts from various disciplines and including international support.

2. Situational analysis starting with field activities (July 1972–November 1972)—a relatively short stage, but comprising extensive field observation and data collection, the work being carried out mostly by the Project working groups in consultation with the Institute of Public Health Research and the School of Public Health of the University of Teheran.

3. Formulation of proposals for plans for further health services development (November 1972–April 1973)—with data processing, consultations, consideration of plans, and attempts to involve wider circles of Project

participants (technical collaborators of participating agencies and organizations, field health workers in the province, and relevant experts in the Ministry of Health).

4. "Preparatory step" (July 1973–March 1974)—feasibility studies, small field trials, detailed planning, starting experimental small-scale action (training and practice of primary health workers in the field), and forming new types of working groups (comprising local health workers, Project participants from the University, and consultants).

5. Implementation (from April 1974 onwards)—including evaluation—with increasing responsibility on the part of the Programme Director (the Provincial Director-General of Health) and the local staff; during implementation there is an urgent need to extrapolate local features to the national level and extend activities into areas not covered.

The Project is planned and conducted as a joint action-oriented research activity. The active participants in the Project include the Ministry of Health, the Red Lion and Sun Society, the Imperial Organization for Social Services, the Social Insurance Organization, the Plan and Budget Organization, and the School of Public Health and Institute of Public Health Research of the University of Teheran, in collaboration with the World Health Organization.

The province of West Azerbaijan—a typical province as regards health conditions—was chosen as the field area for the Project and its Director-General of Health was appointed Programme Director of the Project. He collaborates closely with the Scientific Director of the Project, who is Professor of Public Health Administration at the School of Public Health of the University of Teheran. They are both responsible to a technical Executive Committee of the Project and to a National Committee organized and led by the Ministry of Health and consisting of representatives of the main agencies providing health services for the population.

The West Azerbaijan Project is one example of several projects in Iran aiming at similar goals, including projects organized by the Imperial Organization for Social Services and the Pahlavi University of Shiraz.

Situational analysis

Field area

The province of West Azerbaijan, one of the country's 21 provinces, is in the north-west corner of Iran and has mountains suitable for cattle breeding, fertile plains, cold winters, and difficult communications. Of its 1.3 million inhabitants, about one million live in more than 3300 scattered villages (see Fig. 1). The province is agricultural and there are several projects in operation to increase agricultural production through new irrigation schemes and the organization of rural corporations and co-operatives.

The estimated crude birth rate is high (42–45 per 1000 population) and the estimated crude mortality rate is 10–14 per 1000 population. The

FIG. 1. DISTRIBUTION OF URBAN AND RURAL POPULATION IN WEST AZERBAIJAN

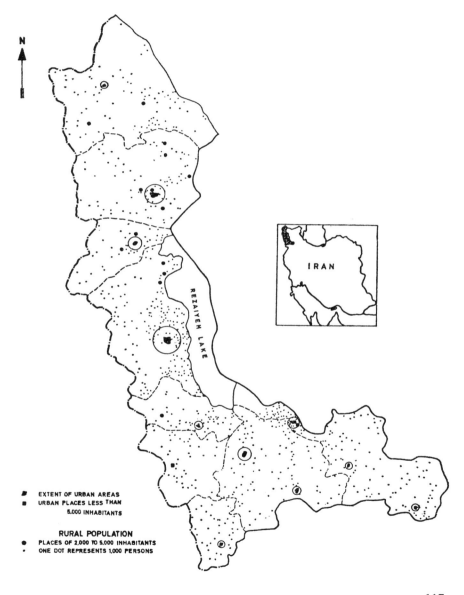

N

IRAN

REZAIYEH LAKE

■ EXTENT OF URBAN AREAS
■ URBAN PLACES LESS THAN
    5,000 INHABITANTS

RURAL POPULATION
● PLACES OF 2,000 TO 5,000 INHABITANTS
· ONE DOT REPRESENTS 1,000 PERSONS

117

results of the census indicate a crude annual population growth of 3.2% in rural areas. There are differences between the urban and rural populations, but the problem of high fertility and population growth is common to both.

The geographical distribution of the existing health services is such that the basic units form a network, with a major health centre in the capital, health centres (where they are developed) in the districts, and units of lower level in the local urban and rural settings. However, these units are parts of different organizations and agencies and their management and supervision are organized through separate channels, the Provincial Director-General of Health having an overall supervisory function.

Personnel are concentrated in the towns and in the three more developed districts, and private practitioners are also concentrated in bigger towns. In September 1974 the physician/population ratio in the province was 1:8000, with a large variation between the urban and rural areas.

The relationship between traditional and modern medicine

A concern for health is part of traditional Iranian culture and has long been evident in the way in which health needs have been felt and met among the population. Healers, herbalists, bone-setters, traditional midwives, priests, wise men, and others are actively engaged in helping the community in connexion with birth, death, invalidity, and suffering. For instance, one of the basic concepts in Avicenna's work, the importance of a balance between "hot" and "cold" in the development of disease, is highly developed and is invoked in everyday life. In heart diseases of the aged, for example, which by nature are "cold", different kinds of "hot" distilled herbs are applied. Such beliefs have been extended to modern medical practices; for example, an injection is usually considered to be "hot", and a vitamin B_{12} injection is believed to cure a "cold" anaemia as well as cleanse the blood.

Knowledge of traditional health practices is propagated by health workers in nearly every village, the best known being those working near shrines, hot springs, and bazaars. At these places are found specialists in three major fields: spiritual sufferings and needs, the treatment of bodily diseases, and skilled "surgical" activities (dentistry, midwifery, and bone-setting).

Modern medicine has penetrated the rural areas together with other developments such as better communications, nutrition, and water supplies, and has usually been introduced in the form of a mass campaign (malaria eradication, vaccination, or family planning). But besides killing flies and mosquitos it has brought the community relief from pain and fever. Even though modern medicine may have proved its efficacy in the eyes of the community, it is still considered as a last resort, when traditional efforts fail. There is not always mutual understanding between the people and health services and at present there is a gap between modern medicine as applied in practice and the expectations of the population. For example, the survey data show that the specific complaint translated as "heart palpitation"—occurring mainly in middle-aged women—often conceals some other complaints that cannot easily be communicated to male doctors.

Analysis of health needs

The Project's situational analysis focused on the processes resulting in the satisfying of the population's needs and demands in the field of health. All organized health services were included, regardless of the type, level, agency, or economic sector. Current practices in traditional medicine and sectors other than health were considered but not extensively studied.

Existing health service data as well as field survey results were used to describe the process of satisfying health needs and demands from three points of view—those of the people (sociological and anthropological studies), existing organized services (operational studies), and epidemiology (medical surveys in the field).

The most obvious characteristic of the picture given by situational analysis was that only a small proportion of health problems was being dealt with by health services activities, especially in the rural areas.

Against this background an attempt was made to classify health needs in such a way as to enable the planning of health services to be structured according to the form of intervention. Three types of health need were distinguished:

1. Mass and emergency problems—here, organized mass campaigns are the most appropriate intervention and the formation of mobile units is an efficient operational programme.

2. The problems of risk groups in the population—here, both an organized community approach and a family approach are necessary, with continuous care for the individual.

3. Illnesses randomly distributed in the community—here, an individual approach is required, i.e., the treatment of episodes of illnesses.

The situational analysis indicated that problems of the first type were well under control in West Azerbaijan. In contrast, the problems of the second type were estimated to be increasing and subject to the least control, coverage by organized services being low and non-selective (amounting to only 20% of the need in a few select urban areas). The demand for treatment of conditions in the third group was also increasing.

Analysis of existing health services

The demands and needs of the population having been classified and described, it was then necessary to consider another component of the process under study—the delivery system. An examination of existing organized health services was made from inventory reports, supplemented by direct observations.

The delivery system as a whole must be considered as functioning at something less than an optimal level. This suboptimal performance can be described in terms of "external" and "internal" factors. The "external" factors include the disproportion between the population's needs and the services available to the population, utilization depending on place of residence, social class, sex, and the accessibility of the service. The greatest disproportion is found in the case of services for the lower social classes in towns and for rural mountain populations. Young children and old people have relatively less access to services. Furthermore, there is a marked variation in the coverage achieved by the various kinds of services, the coverage for medical needs, especially in adult men, being greatest and that for some exclusively preventive services, e.g., services for pregnant women, being very narrow.

Certain "internal" technical and organizational factors have accentuated the less than optimal functioning of existing services. Among these is the importance attributed to the role of the physician, especially in rural services. Consequently there is a discontinuity of service in small units, which must stop work when the physician is not present, a situation that occurs quite frequently as a result of the high turn-over of physicians, their scarcity relative to available posts, competition between agencies, and the lack of a standardized pattern of work.

The referral rates are generally very low for the system as a whole and even for units within the same agency. This is an expression of the isolated environment within which health units must work. It also indicates that all units are working at about the same technical level.

The approach to health services development

Principles of the approach

A vast number of technically viable solutions exists for improving the delivery system. However, the experience of other delivery systems in similar situations shows that many of these "solutions" are not feasible, especially those requiring the use of improved technology. It was therefore proposed that the main stimulus for initiating and propagating the development of the delivery system in the West Azerbaijan Project should come from within the existing services, and specifically from their inter-

120

action with the population and society; in practice, this meant making the process of health services development operational.

Development implies change. If the change is not to be imposed from the outside, it must be one that is managed from within. The first steps towards development should be clearly defined and should act as a stimulus to the "managers" of the system to direct subsequent changes towards the more efficient attainment of the planned health objectives. So that this process can be realized, a number of supporting steps must be implemented. First, mechanisms must be established for developing operational standards, evaluating their applicability and appropriateness, and improving the health technology applied. Secondly, there must be a concomitant building of communications and improved decision-making to ensure that these mechanisms are being utilized properly. Thirdly, whatever technological changes are introduced must be supported by the rest of the delivery system.

This concept of managed change became the Project's foundation, upon which it was possible to introduce new functions into the system and permit the necessary adjustments to be made so that these functions could be fully realized. In particular, primary health care functions at the village level were introduced by the use of new types of primary health workers, whose role is described below.

Primary health workers as entry points to the system

In a large village near the Rezaiyeh lake there is a health centre operated by the Health Corps, serving the 30 000 inhabitants of about 90 villages, some of which have *khaneh behdasht* (health posts), which were established during the preparatory step of the Project. The way in which the *khaneh behdasht* was set up is typical of *khaneh behdasht* in the province. After part of a rural house had been cleaned and repaired, three of its rooms were simply equipped as a waiting room, a room for health workers, and a consultation room. In the nearby garden a latrine was built.

The *behyar mama rustai* (rural nurse/midwife) operates from the *khaneh behdasht*. These nurses are recruited from the village housing the *khaneh behdasht* or from nearby villages, in collaboration with the local population. They are young women, but not younger than 16, preferably with 6 years of primary schooling. They have to carry out a programme covering the functions of a health "mother": care for children, help in ailments, simple treatment, referrals, and first aid in specified cases. Their work is divided between home visits, especially those relating to small children and infants, and work at the consultation room, where they work alone or with supervisors and a doctor once a fortnight.

Part of their work is done together with their neighbouring *behyar mama rustai* and with a *behdasht yar* (male health worker)—a former participant in malaria eradication programmes, a retrained member of other health or epidemiological teams, or a sanitary technician. They work together, for instance, in vaccination programmes and some aspects of family planning programmes. The *behdasht yar* is the health "father" of the groups. At present he is concerned not so much with providing personal care for patients as with organizing and supporting the activities of the *behyar mama rustai* and, particularly, taking part in health campaigns and organizing the community to keep the village clean and healthy. He is mobile and closely connected with the health centre, which houses his immediate supervisor. In the field his responsibility extends over a territory equalling that of two *khaneh behdasht* (a total population of 5000–7000).

The *behyar mama rustai* is not competing for work with indigenous midwives in villages; she provides an additional part of prenatal care, early screening for hospital delivery, and care for newborns.

Of the first reported 1000 contacts in *khaneh behdasht*, about 600 related to particular complaints or repeated treatment procedures and the remainder to mothers and children with or without complaints but included in active screening, education, nutrition, or treatment programmes.

FIG. 2. PROPOSED ORGANIZATION OF HEALTH SERVICES IN WEST AZERBAIJAN.

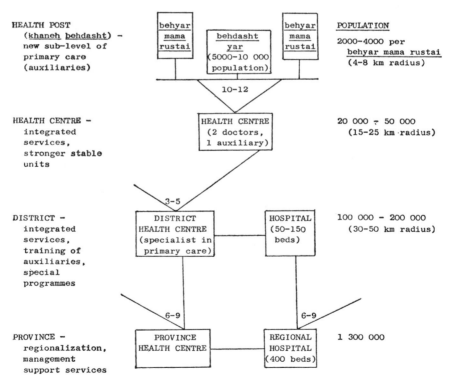

122

The *behdasht yar* continued carrying out the tasks of a malaria surveillance worker but his work load in that programme was diminished by one-third. Instead he carries out additional tasks in connexion with vaccination, screening, the maintenance of environmental sanitation facilities, and other community health actions.

The organizational setting in which the two new types of primary health workers function is shown in Fig. 2. The *behyar mama rustai* and the *behdasht yar* are able to refer problems that are beyond their present capabilities to the health centre, which has the first doctor contact. Subsequently, the doctor and centre will be able to use skills and services more appropriate to a health centre structure, i.e., a level of health care different from that provided by the new primary health workers and also from the present front line of care.

The same concept applies to the remaining contacts of care. When a health centre, through lack of the necessary skills or techniques, is unable to provide a particular kind of medical care (curative or preventive), the problem is referred to the next higher level. At the district level there is a specialist in community health needs and facilities for providing secondary care—outpatient services and a small hospital. If these facilities are inadequate, the problem can be referred to the provincial hospital, where a range of specialists handle more complex medical care needs or transfer patients to the "national level".

The training of the *behyar mama rustai* and *behdasht yar* is already in progress but its final stages are still being planned. They start work in the villages after a few weeks of basic training and are expected to continue to work intermittently and to attend classes for 2 years; for this reason they are doubled in every post at the beginning. They are trained in one of the schools for health auxiliaries in the province. Their training is mostly practical: they are taught how to carry out well-defined procedures, how to understand people, and how to collaborate with traditional health workers and laymen.

The training is based on the development of standard tasks in order to ensure the consistency and quality of work at the primary level. First, they are instructed in a number of procedures relating to the most frequent health needs and demands where effective treatment can be found. A described procedure contains specific tasks and steps the health workers have to follow. Of a total of 23 tasks designed for the *behdasht yar*, 3 relate to malaria eradication programmes, 4 to the tuberculosis programme, 4 to immunization, 5 to environmental sanitation, and the rest to several other activities (first aid, etc.). The *behyar mama rustai* was initially charged with 16 tasks in active care for mothers and children and in the family planning programme. There are also 16 tasks in the field of medical care, starting with most frequent complaints. Altogether there are about 80 initially defined elementary parts of different tasks, such as filling in a child health card, weighing infants, giving an intramuscular injection of diphtheria/pertussis/tetanus vaccine, and sterilizing instruments by boiling.

The main aim is to extend the coverage by means of simple and effective procedures using as much of the existing patterns and resources as possible. The total activities are expected to ensure that 90% of households will be visited according to the requirements of the malaria eradication surveillance programme and that at least 80% of the eligible population will receive the vaccines included in the national immunization programme. The *khaneh behdasht* staff will be responsible for introducing and maintaining improvements in environmental sanitation for at least half the villages that are not at present covered. They will also collect baseline demographic data in not less than 90% of households. They will ensure mother and child care for at least 80% of the target population and family planning coverage for at least 60% of eligible women. It is expected that the *khaneh behdasht* staff will attend 10% of deliveries and handle directly two-thirds of the complaints presented.

Several other distributions of tasks and procedures are foreseen; e.g., for remote areas with very small villages and difficult communications the role of the *behdasht yar* should be widened to include more first-aid and treatment procedures. The same applies to procedures conditioned by different types of local morbidity: instead of the tuberculosis programme, another programme might be covered, e.g., endemic syphilis, trachoma, or leprosy.

A similar scheme was to be implemented in towns, but first in poorly developed areas, the medical care component of the primary health workers' duties being concentrated in centres and clinics, under supervision and in consultation with physicians.

The present situation

Evaluation of the activities of the preparatory step described above has shown that the new types of primary health workers have been integrated into the health services system as well as into the community, in the experimental area, during the first year of operations. Although the training of the primary health workers has not yet been completed, they have been able to carry out the specified tasks. Their work is already reflected in a considerable fall in the number of patients coming to see the physician in the rural health centre from areas covered by the primary health workers.

Special attention has been paid to the management aspects of the system. Regular supervision of the primary health workers is carried out by the staff of the rural health centre, mainly the physician. The primary health workers can refer patients to the rural health centre with which they are associated.

124

In the light of the experience gained during the preparatory step, the introduction of primary health workers was started in the late spring of 1974 in three districts of the West Azerbaijan by personnel of the Ministry of Health. Following a course to train the trainers, a course is being conducted in each of the three districts to train the first groups of primary health workers to function under non-experimental conditions. As evaluation is considered to be an important mechanism in the further development of the scheme, the progress of the implementation is closely monitored so that information may be obtained for the extension of the project to other districts of the province and later to other provinces.

Discussion

Integration with the social system and other health services

The *khaneh behdasht* cannot exist without support from both the local community and from other services in the community. They also need the acceptance and support of the health services themselves and of other health practitioners.

A prerequisite for the successful role of the primary health worker was considered to be a well-defined but flexible job description. Referral and regular supervision had to be adequately thought out in practical operational terms.

The job description was considered in terms of medical and health procedures for front-line services, with a view to strengthening the remaining components of the delivery system. For example, estimates were made of the structure and load of referral cases, from which decisions could be made on how best to meet these needs and the anticipated impact on the other existing services. From operational assumptions and calculations it was proposed that one health centre or clinic could support 8–12 *khaneh behdasht*; from this organizational starting-point it was possible to define the personnel and management requirements for this level of services.

From the situational analysis—on the basis of existing and projected resources—the expected number of operating health centres in rural areas could also be estimated. From these estimates it was concluded that the rural health centre network should not be extended but that the centres should be strengthened at selected points. In addition, it was proposed that this rural network should be actively supported by the next (district) level of health centres.

Districts are formed around small towns and trade and social centres, usually with a small hospital and a district health centre. The district is the lowest level currently considered to be capable of attracting and retaining physicians for more than two years. Therefore, the proposal for West Azerbaijan put great emphasis on the district level of health services. The district is planned to provide support to the rural health centres where the mostly young and inexperienced physicians work, to be responsible for supervision and the first review of field data, and to act as a coordinating centre for the training of primary health workers.

A suitably oriented medical man is required to manage and guide the district level of service. Therefore, it was further proposed that a specific postgraduate training programme should be started, based on existing patterns of courses leading to the degree of Master in Public Health but aiming at specialization in professionally recognized, comprehensive, primary care.

Summary of operational aspects

The proposal for strengthening the health services delivery system of West Azerbaijan can be summarized by outlining the specific operational objectives of the plan. In the area of primary care the objectives include: the development of front-line health posts (*khaneh behdasht*) housing two new types of primary health worker (the *behyar mama rustai* and the *behdasht yar*), the strengthening of the doctor/health-centre level of primary care to ensure a continuous service, the integration of essential curative components of care into active preventive services, and the improvement of the training and management capabilities of the district level units. The following objectives were formulated for the further levels of care: reorganization of hospital outpatient units to function at a referral–care level, and regionalization of hospitals to provide more coordination of functions and support. These two changes must also be supported by the management improvements identified earlier: the introduction of management mechanisms, the strengthening of the communication and decision-making processes, and the alteration of supporting services to ensure the technical viability of these changes.

Expectations for the future

The necessity of developing a new line of primary health services might be questioned if the rapid development of the country could permit primary and other care to be provided by staff who have undergone a longer education. It would perhaps be more profitable to concentrate on isolated, highly developed units and expect the broader population group to reach and utilize services at that contact point. Two factors must be taken into account in this regard. First, the development of a new line of primary care is not a measure to replace other parts but a step towards building a bridge between the population and the services; the formal application of measures incorporating apparently high-quality medical care is not necessarily a step forward in improving the health status of the population. The second point is that isolated, highly developed units, even where heavily utilized, may not be able to provide a basis for covering the total population in the future; they could suffer the same social rejection that other units have experienced and, as a consequence, would have to be excluded from any future plan.

The introduction of a new primary contact is an inexpensive stimulating measure bringing the challenge of the most frequent health problems of the population to comprehensive multidisciplinary and technically developed medicine. The resources necessary to build that bridge with the population are less expensive than any other part of the system and the influence could be profound and far-reaching.

Will that type of system be acceptable after 20 years? Substantial changes can come with a successful break-through in technology. However, there are three factors that affect the acceptability of the system even after such a long period.

First, even with essential social changes in the population structure, population growth will mean that the rural segment remains as large in absolute numbers, or even increases.

The second factor is flexibility of the planned system. It is likely that the level of education of the front-line workers will be increasingly higher, but health needs will continue to be best understood by people in close contact with those needs. In other words, the front line should develop with the population.

The third factor is the experience in some developed countries of the need to use auxiliary personnel. The nature of the health problems is changing, so that changes in education and procedures are needed, but underlying needs for personal health care and follow-up continue and even increase. A good example of such changing needs is seen in a developed society with problems of chronic diseases and mental diseases.

The experience of many countries is that hospitals and medical schools have a far-reaching influence on the development of health services; the regional system described needs to be supplemented with adequate changes at the highest level, including research and professional education. However, before all the elements can be defined the system has to show that it is capable of developing internal cooperation through standardization of procedures, joint in-service training, unified technical supervision, and a coordinated information system. Since the health services system may be regarded as in transition, fixed structures and a unified command do not of themselves solve problems.

VILLAGE HEALTH TEAMS IN NIGER (MARADI DEPARTMENT)

G. FOURNIER & I.A. DJERMAKOYE [a]

The Republic of Niger has, for a number of years, relied on voluntary workers to cover the elementary health needs of populations living in remote areas. These voluntary health workers are chosen by the village communities and participate actively in curative as well as preventive care activities.

The following account of the results obtained by applying this method in the Maradi Department, Niger, shows that this is a valuable approach to the solution of problems caused by the chronic lack of health personnel.

General information on the Maradi Department

Relatively privileged compared with the rest of Niger, the Department of Maradi, with a surface of about 38 500 km², is situated in the central part of the country along the Nigerian frontier, half-way between the Niger River to the West and Lake Chad to the East. For administrative purposes the Department is divided into 6 counties *(arrondissements)* and one municipality (Maradi). The road network is rather poor. Of the 730 000 inhabitants, 95% are engaged in agricultural activities in the south; in the north, where the population density is low, there is extensive livestock farming.

The Maradi Department is in the northern part of the Sudan area of very sparsely wooded savanna. There are only a few intermittent rivers *(goulbi)* and a large permanent pool (Lake Madarounfa). The ground water layers, which feed wells 40–80 metres deep, are therefore the region's main water resources.

The water supply for the majority of the rural population is drawn either from ponds (permanent or temporary) or wells, in most cases contaminated as a result of primitive drawing methods. In general, people defaecate directly on to the ground around dwellings—cesspits,

[a] In collaboration with M. Torfs, Division of Strengthening of Health Services, World Health Organization, Geneva, Switzerland.

latrines, and septic tanks are rare and in most cases unused. There are no sanitary installations in most of the villages and they are rare in towns.

Morbidity and mortality are very high, particularly among children: the general mortality rate is estimated at 27 per 1000, whereas the infant mortality rate lies between 250 and 300 per 1000 live births; only 40% of children reach the age of 5 years. Of the persons attending the health establishments of the Department as a whole, 35% are under 5 years of age, whereas that age group constitutes only 17% of the population.

The main diseases are infectious or parasitic and their incidence could be easily decreased by better hygiene. For example, conjunctivitis and infections of the skin and mouth account for 25% of consultations, while malaria (falciparum) and enteritis account for 26%. Chest complaints, tuberculous and otherwise, are also very frequent (18%). To these illnesses must be added venereal disease, particularly in the north (among nomads) and the towns, as well as illnesses related to pregnancy and childbirth, which are very frequent and result in high morbidity and mortality among pregnant women and newborn babies.

Regular vaccination campaigns have resulted in the disappearance of smallpox and have considerably decreased the incidence of measles. Cerebro-spinal meningitis is prevalent during the dry season to an extent that varies from year to year. Leprosy is of little significance and urinary bilharziasis is limited to the areas around infected pools.

Infant malnutrition is widespread and appears towards the age of 8–10 months, as has been shown by study of the infant weights recorded in all the dispensaries of the Department. It regresses towards the age of 4–5 years and is mainly protein-calorie malnutrition of the wasting type or incomplete forms of kwashiorkor. The absence of frank kwashiorkor, combined with the fact that malnutrition is accompanied by numerous infections or parasitoses, explains why it is rarely taken into consideration by the nurses and is not included in the periodic reports of the different health establishments.

This protein-calorie malnutrition is caused by inadequate feeding practices; either the infant receives only its mother's milk or, once weaned, is given only millet gruel prepared with water and very undercooked. Thus, the high mortality and morbidity mainly among children is explained by poor hygiene combined with malnutrition, both these factors being related to ignorance and socioeconomic conditions.

The following infrastructure operates under the direction and super-vision of the departmental health services: a departmental hospital with 139 beds, a departmental mobile team for health and hygiene, an urban maternal and child health centre and a dispensary in Maradi, and 6 health areas *(circonscriptions médicales d'arrondissements)*. The latter have a total of 17 rural dispensaries, 3 medical centres with a total of 82 beds, and 4 maternity units with a total of 38 beds. The bed/population ratio is about 1:6000 if the urban health services covering Maradi municipality are not taken into consideration. However, it has been decided to enlarge this infrastructure during the period of the next five-year plan (1975–1979) by the construction of a rural dispensary, 3 medical centres with a total of 60 beds, and 3 maternity units with a total of 24 beds.

The participation of the private sector (missions) in the functioning of health services is limited to one leprosarium and one rural dispensary. The health personnel working in the public sector comprise 8 medical officers, 1 dentist, 3 midwives, 24 state registered nurses, 57 nurses, and 16 auxiliary nurses—giving a ratio of one medical officer for 230 000 population and one nurse or auxiliary nurse for 12 300 inhabitants in rural areas. A rural dispensary normally covers the area within a radius of 10–15 km. With one dispensary for about 30 000 inhabitants, one maternity unit per 175 000 population, and with the uneven distribution of personnel, the fixed health service is too weak and too much limited to the main towns and large villages to be able to respond adequately to the health needs of the whole population. Moreover, the mobile team for health and hygiene, which carries out vaccinations and case-finding in all the villages of the Department every 3 years, can have only a transitory effect on the rural population's health.

Thus the health establishments of the Department as a whole cover less than 15% of patients, so that 85% of the sick are treating themselves or are being treated by traditional healers, with all the consequent risks. Quite apart from this inadequacy of manpower and facilities, the personnel, who do not usually originate from the locality where they work, tend to be ignorant of local public health problems, their training and outlook being oriented towards curative medicine. Although serious efforts have been made in the past few years to incorporate public health concepts into the nurses' training, any knowledge of preventive medicine—when it exists—remains purely theoretical, while maternal and child care, health education, and sanitation rarely form part of the day-to-day activities of the nurses.

Moreover, the few rare and rapid tours of the bush made by the more zealous doctors and nurses are often ineffective, so difficult, if not impossible, is contact between an urban official who arrives unrequested and a peasant who merely sees him come and go. This frequent absence of dialogue and understanding leads sometimes to dispensaries that have been constructed spontaneously by the villagers being found several years afterwards in ruins, for they have never been used owing to the lack of a nurse and equipment.

The original health situation may therefore be summarized as follows. First, there was a high morbidity and mortality resulting from poor hygiene and malnutrition. Secondly, there was a health service network whose mesh was too large and whose personnel often restricted themselves to purely curative activities for the benefit of the urban population only.

Finally, dialogue appeared impossible between a rural population that did not know how to express its requirements and a health service not prepared to acknowledge and respond to them.

The basic approach used: extension work

However, for some years it has seemed possible to narrow or even eliminate this gap between the health services and the rural population by bringing them together so that they can cooperate to ensure permanent and effective health protection at the village level.

The first experiments in Niger were made in 1963, when at Tillaberi (Niamey Department) and Matameye (Zinder Department) the rural health and extension services trained village health workers (*secouristes-hygiénistes*) to be responsible for giving treatment and developing hygiene in villages distant from any dispensary.

A year afterwards, taking into account these initial experiments, the Ministry of Health set out in the *Ten-Year Prospects—1965-1974*, and then in the *Quadrennial Plans—1965-1968 and 1971-1974*, the aims and principles that should govern the training of such auxiliaries.

The training of a village health worker will enable him to carry out the routine cleaning and dressing of wounds and to administer simple medicaments, and will facilitate hygiene measures and the cooperation of the population in mass health service campaigns. This training will be given in close cooperation with the rural extension services and will lead to the local community assuming responsibility for public health. As a rule, these village health workers will be volunteers. The village community will make itself responsible for renewal of the standard village pharmacy kit. The village health worker will be appointed by the village and will have to bear a certain responsibility... General awareness (as regards suitable health attitudes and habits) will be ensured by a constant informational and educational effort carried on by a village team (village health workers, traditional birth attendants) acting as permanent representatives of the health service...
Activities (health and dietetic education) will be carried on by ... the village health workers.. Traditional birth attendants and village health workers will be supervised by the nurses of medical centres, or medical counties, and by the physician in charge of the departmental mobile teams.

However, no systematic development of village health workers and traditional birth attendants was organized at that time in the Departments and these auxiliaries came into being only on the occasion of personal and limited contacts between a few doctors, nurses, and rural extension officials.

Thus, in the Maradi Department, there was a succession of isolated experiments—village health workers and traditional birth attendants at Maradi in 1966 and village health workers at Tessaoua in 1967 and at Dakoro in 1968. Subsequently, in 1970, thanks to concerted action and to exchanges between the health personnel of the Departments, the various experiments were integrated so that the training of village health workers and traditional birth attendants could be organized and gradually extended throughout the Department (even in regions without extension workers). This organized development is the original feature of the achievements in the Maradi Department.

As a result, on 1 January 1974 Niger had 780 village health workers in 362 villages (including 216 in 108 villages of the Maradi Department) and 467 village midwives in 179 villages (including 266 in 88 Maradi villages). To mobilize the health personnel and population in this way, extension techniques have had to be used, which consist in getting everyone to participate in the common task by making them individually aware of their responsibility in the community.

Extension work among the rural population

Since 1963 the rural extension services *(animation rurale)* in the Republic of Niger have existed in the form of community development schemes characterized by the voluntary participation of the population and their active responsibility in socioeconomic development; these schemes combine, within the framework of national development, the structures and the efforts of the communities with those of the technical services. For this reason the rural extension services form part of the administrative structure at all levels (local, departmental, and national), like the other technical services, to which they bring their support by educating and motivating the village community.

Within that framework and for more than 10 years now in the Department of Maradi, the rural extension services (employing both men and women) have enabled the peasants, thanks to persistent surveys and efforts to arouse their awareness, to express long-felt health needs that they could not previously have expressed because of the lack of any real and continuing contact with the health services. Population groups have been shown how they can participate in health activities directly concerning their village.

By means of contacts, first individual and then increasingly official, the rural extension services have led the health services to take an active part in carrying on activities in the villages with the aim of setting up peasant teams (village health workers and traditional birth attendants) at the village level, responsible for promoting health by dealing with immediate curative needs and by developing hygiene.

Although this mobilization of the rural population remains fragmentary, since the rural extension services cover only a small part of the Department and the country, it has gradually become evident that the active participation of the peasants in protecting their health at the village level could be an effective aid to the official services in this field, always provided that doctors and nurses agree to play their part in the same spirit and to go beyond the walls of the dispensaries, which are devoted solely to curative treatment.

In this way, even in areas not covered by extension services, nurses have been able, together with the population, to undertake real rural health extension work. Since these activities were in some cases too dependent upon the personality of individuals, they have temporarily failed because of lack of continuity. It would therefore seem essential to carry on extension work among the health personnel parallel with that among the rural population.

Extension work in the health service

For nearly four years, extension work in the health service has been undertaken in the Maradi Department, in close cooperation with the rural extension and literacy services. This action has consisted, on the one hand, of bringing the personnel as a whole (whatever their level) to consider themselves responsible not merely for a dispensary or a particular service but for the whole population to be served, and, on the other hand, has encouraged the same personnel to practise *global medicine*, comprising care, prevention, health education, and the collection of medical, social, and economic information.

It is interesting to note that such extension work among the health personnel, like that among the rural population, calls for research, reflection, and dialogue on the part of all the participants. Thus, the health situation described above is gradually becoming known. At the outset, since the nurses were used to playing a very passive role, there was no motivation for them to wonder about the health situation of their village or region. However, an initial approach is being made by the use of statistical reports. The examination of these reports (never previously used in the field) makes the nurses realize the value of their work and encourages them to collect other data by engaging in new activities, such as maternal and child health, that they had previously refused. The health impact of the dispensaries, malnutrition, and infant morbidity has been assessed in this way, and there is greater awareness of these public health problems. During the quarterly district and departmental study meetings, this information is exchanged and short-term plans of work established, after discussions between the different participants: prefect or sub-prefect, doctors and nurses, and those responsible for rural extension, literacy, and education. Since they call for the nurses to prepare concrete and precise descriptions or reports of activities that are discussed by all participants, these meetings lead to great emulation between them and constitute a veritable training school. The authorities and other services rapidly took a very keen interest in the meetings, where frankness and realism have always prevailed, thus making productive teamwork possible. The meetings are supplemented by refresher courses, where epidemiology and prevention are emphasized in addition to treatment, which remains realistic and takes into account the facilities available in the dispensaries and villages.

The implementation of the approach

Thus, thanks to the use of extension techniques, it has been possible to set up health teams consisting of village health workers and traditional birth attendants, trained and supported by the health personnel and the rural extension and literacy services (where these exist).

Village health workers

The village health workers are the representatives of the health service at the village level, responsible for organizing protection against epidemic diseases (isolation, notification, assistance in vaccination campaigns), improving hygiene and sanitation, and giving simple treatment for common diseases, using a kit containing certain basic drugs. This curative activity seems to correspond best to the needs felt by the population and always takes precedence over the others, to such an extent that the team of village health workers is popularly known as the "village pharmacy", the term which is used in this account although it may at first sight seem too restrictive. The personnel of the village pharmacy are peasant volunteers —normally two village health workers aided by a "management committee" consisting of the chairman and the treasurer of the pharmacy.

The village health workers are directly responsible for care and hygiene in the village. One of them keeps a treatment record book in which all treatment given is noted daily. The chairman and treasurer enter in an account book the money received for those drugs that have to be paid for. They renew supplies as the need arises from the "Popular Pharmacy" of the district capital town, either directly or through the nurse of the nearest dispensary or the chief of the medical district. Both are involved in the supervision of the activities. Apart from individual and friendly arrangements, the only compensation for the work accomplished by the village health worker consists, in theory, of assistance from the villagers, who work in his fields or gardens.

The drugs and other products made available to the village health workers are characterized by effectiveness, ease of handling, and modest cost, and are provided to combat the main diseases encountered in the region. In order to avoid wastage and to lessen the financial burden on the districts, products in the form of tablets must be paid for. In this way, the village health workers can treat nearly 50% of patients in their village with: soap and mercurochrome, for wounds and skin conditions; methylene blue, for oral infections; silver proteinate eye-drops, for conjunctivitis; sulfaguanidine (against payment), for infective diarrhoea; and amodiaquine or chloroquine (against payment), for malaria (amodiaquine is often preferred because it can be prescribed in a single curative and preventive dose). To these basic drugs are sometimes added: gomenol, ethanolic solutions of boric acid, aureomycin eye ointment, and aspirin.

In one typical village the community has built a straw hut enclosed by a small fence, to facilitate the work of the village health workers. Every morning the patients receive their care here. Mamadou, a young village health worker recently returned from his training period, cleans the wounds and instils eye drops into the eyes of a few patients. Nearby, Issaka gives three tablets of amodiaquine to Hadiza to cure her presumptive malaria attack. Issaka has now been a village health worker for two years and this year attended the literacy course; he therefore records in his notebook all the care given during the day. In the afternoon he gives to Ibrahim, the treasurer, the money received from Hazida as payment for her tablets. In the afternoon Issaka and Mamadou are called from their fields because Idi has seriously injured his foot with his *daba* (hoe). After cleansing and dressing the wound Issaka refers the patient to the nearest dispensary (about 18 km away) and Mamadou is to accompany the patient, who has been installed on horseback.

When villages are being chosen as locations for setting up pharmacies, account is taken of the wishes of the population, as well as the geographical, economic, social, and health conditions; accordingly, the choice is made in cooperation with the administrative and political authorities and those responsible for the various district services.

It is essential, in fact, to take full account of the conditions under which the monthly supervision that these new village pharmacies impose on the nurses of the rural clinics can be carried out; the nurses have to make their supervisory tours on horseback, and the number of village pharmacies established should not be too large to permit regular inspection. Most failures are caused by the village health workers being left to themselves, when their willingness becomes exhausted in the absence of moral, technical, and logistic support.

The village health workers, chairman and treasurer are chosen by the villagers from volunteers, if possible literate ones. Since the choice governs the success of the operation, it is essential for the village populations to understand perfectly the aims and the functions of a pharmacy and the part played by each person; for this reason, an intensive attempt to arouse their awareness should precede any training or refresher courses for village health workers.

Thus, at an early stage, after arranging an interview with the village chief and influential persons and carefully explaining their purpose and procedure, the responsible extension and health officials organize one or more meetings attended by all the villagers, the village chief, the *iman* and his *marabouts*, merchants, the head of the canton, and the Sub-Prefect (or their representatives). After the introduction of the participants, a general survey is made of the topic of health—frequency of illnesses, inadequacy of the dispensaries, nurses, and transport, difficulty in transporting patients and in making notifications of disease, loss of time and expense involved in going to the dispensary to have minor illnesses treated. During this initial discussion, the responsible officials take into account the social and health enquiry that should have been made on the preceding days to enable the villagers to express their views more easily.

The creation of a village pharmacy and the training of volunteers to ensure its proper functioning is then proposed. During the discussion, everything should be explained in detail: the aim and functioning of the pharmacy; the roles of the village health workers, the chairman, and the treasurer; the fees for drugs and the method of supply; the date, duration, and place of training courses; and the means of transport and maintenance of trainees. Finally, the main criteria for choosing the village health workers are defined: they must be volunteers and, if possible, literate; they must be adults and attached to the village; they must not travel too much; they must be honest, loved, and respected by all; and they must be patient and discreet.

After 8-10 days a further meeting takes place during which the villagers introduce the village health workers, the chairman, and the treasurer they have chosen. The details of the training course and any points still obscure are then clarified.

The annual training and refresher training courses take place at the rural dispensary that serves as the base for the work. The courses must not exceed 7–10 days in length, since the peasants do not like to remain too long away from their village—7 days of medical instruction and 3 days of literacy training and book-keeping work. The programme must obviously not be overloaded and should impart only simple, practical, and precise knowledge that can be immediately put to use. The training programme includes hygiene, elementary and emergency care, health and nutritional education, and instruction on how to make records of patients in notebooks. Over the course of the years, the level of knowledge can be built up on the foundation of what has been previously learnt; in this way, subjects such as malnutrition, vaccination, malaria, chemoprophylaxis, and waste disposal can be gradually added.

All training courses must be adapted to the peasant trainees. The theoretical part is short, the brief explanations being interrupted by questions to see how far they have been understood; the simpler the courses the greater the interest shown by the trainees. By means of practical exercises and sketches during the village gatherings, any points that have not been understood can be made clear.

The success of the training also depends, to a large extent, on organization: the trainees should receive a better meal than they usually have,

136

and there should be free time for recreation in the evenings. Relations between instructors and trainees are also very important and should be simple and friendly and avoid the usual barriers between town dwellers and peasants. The instructor therefore tries to live a rural life with the trainees, at the same time enquiring about their needs and their reactions to the courses, meals, and other matters.

For all these reasons, it is necessary for the team responsible for the training (chief of the medical district, nurse of the nearest dispensary, agents of the extension and literacy service) to have participated in the process of preparation and motivation and for the village health workers to see them regularly later on during the periodic inspection visits.

The return of the village health workers to their village is as important a stage in the process of motivation as those that have preceded training. After an absence of some 10 days, the village health workers are generally given a warm reception, just as if they had come back from a long journey. The villagers all come to see what they have brought back, in particular the medicine kit. On this occasion it is advisable to assemble the population, together with the authorities, so that the trainees can explain what they have learnt and again define their role, the aim of the operation, and what they expect from the village (in connexion with the hygiene of the settlements, for example).

Once a month, the village pharmacy is supervised by the nurse from the nearest health establishment. During his visits he evaluates the number of treatments given by the village health workers. Together with them, he examines the patients, giving advice on care, hygiene, nutrition, or evacuation, as necessary. He checks the state of cleanliness of the village with the aim of helping to improve sanitation and general hygiene. Finally, he replenishes the supply of free drugs. The results of the inspection of the village pharmacies for which he is responsible are transmitted every month by the nurse to the chief of the medical district. Every 2–3 months, the latter, together with the responsible rural extension official (in the regions covered by that service), supplements the monthly inspection by checking the smooth running of the pharmacy and its impact on the villagers.

It is often during these inspection visits that any incompetence or unwillingness of a poorly chosen village health worker or the lack of knowledge of the population regarding the functioning of the pharmacy become apparent. It is therefore essential for these checks to be made regularly so that the nurse or the chief of the medical district can continue the training of the village health workers, the chairman, and treasurer, as well as the motivation of the population. It is on this occasion also that the annual refresher courses or new training courses are prepared, for the voluntary village health workers may not wish to continue and may be changed by the village. The distribution of work between the village health workers and the management committee is also sometimes modified at that time.

To summarize, all contacts with the peasants, whether village health workers or not, afford an opportunity to have the pharmacy taken over to an increasing extent by the community, so that every villager can feel personnally involved in its functioning.

Traditional birth attendants

Unlike the case of the village health workers, no new development is involved here, merely an improvement of the function of the traditional midwife *(matrone)* who has always existed in the villages.   These traditional birth attendants play a passive and ritual role, for they are called in only after delivery to cut the cord, bury the placenta, and give some "care" to the mother and child.   Consequently, there is no question of their playing any part in the prevention and early diagnosis of the diseases of pregnancy or childbirth that are responsible for so many maternal and infant deaths.

The operation, at first undertaken around Maradi (1966) and then gradually extended to the whole Department, consists of giving the traditional birth attendants some elementary medical training to enable them to intervene before, during, and after delivery.

For the present, since most of the traditional birth attendants are elderly, only simple principles are taught: detection of oedema; hygiene of the pregnant woman; hygiene of the settlement; delivery on a clean mat (or piece of plasticized linen); evacuation of haemorrhage and unduly long labour cases; ligature, cutting, and dressing of the cord; instilling eye drops in to the eyes of the newborn baby; feeding the newborn baby and infant; giving gruel consisting of millet boiled with milk, or using groundnut cake, from the age of 5 months.

The training courses last 10–15 days and take place in the district maternity clinic under the direction of the midwife (or a nurse) and with the assistance of the women's extension service (if this exists).   The traditional birth attendants participate, during the course, in all the activities of the maternity clinic.   Finally, after a brief examination, those deemed suitable are given a record book, in which they have every birth entered (by a literate person or the *marabout*), and a kit (UNICEF type) containing: plasticized linen, cotton wool, compresses, bandages, merbromin, silver proteinate, ligatures, and razor blades.   Some of these items may be replaced locally from the stocks of the village pharmacy.

The villages that are to receive this service and the traditional birth attendants are selected in much the same way as in the case of the village health workers.   However, it has been found necessary to arrange separate meetings for the women and for the men, and sometimes by sector, since a traditional birth attendant is rarely accepted by everyone; generally she works only for one sector of the village or even a large family.   Younger,

138

and sometimes literate, women may be chosen in place of traditional birth attendants who are too old. In that case, they must have the consent of their husband and that of the women whom they will have to look after.

Thus, the period of motivation is long and preceded by a thorough social and health survey at the village level. Technical inspection is hardly possible in the absence of a qualified midwife or female nurse; therefore, the supervising (male) nurse does no more than record the notifications of birth (which give the right to an official birth certificate) and replenish the stock of products in the kit.

On average, the traditional birth attendants are given refresher courses every two years.

The cost of a village health team

In principle, every dispensary nurse should spend several days every month on medical tours of duty in his canton, just like the chief of the medical district in his district. A travel budget is provided for this purpose and should, therefore, include transport costs for monthly or fortnightly inspection of the village health teams. The cost of the village health workers and midwives programme can therefore be calculated in relation to tours for motivation of the villagers, training or refresher courses, and the provision of kits. The annual maintenance cost of the latter (with the exception of drugs paid for, supplies of which are renewed using the money paid for the drugs by the villagers) is very moderate and easily borne by the working budget for the running of the base dispensary.

The cost of training two village health workers (10-day course) and the chairman and treasurer (3-day course) amounts to Fr. CFA 5200 (Fr. CFA 200 per day), while the pharmacy kit costs about Fr. CFA 6000.[a]

For an average village of 300–400 inhabitants, 3–4 traditional birth attendants are needed; their 15-day training costs Fr. CFA 12 000 and their kit costs Fr. CFA 3000.

Thus, the cost of a village health team during the first year is about Fr. CFA 26 000, to which must be added the cost of the petrol necessary for making 5–6 motivation visits. In subsequent years the cost falls to Fr. CFA 17 000 or even less, since the refresher courses for traditional birth attendants are not annual. There can be no doubt that, taking into account the results obtained, the financial cost is particularly low since it involves only training. In addition, the community frequently builds a straw hut in order to facilitate the care activities.

In practice, although presents have always been given to the traditional birth attendant on the occasion of a birth, the village health workers receive

---

[a] US$1 = Fr. CFA 245; Fr. CFA 1 = US$0.004 (1974).

nothing for the care they give. The villagers should help them to work their fields, since they may be called upon every day and at any time, but this has so far been done only in exceptional cases.

It is not only the mere monetary expense of the village operation that must be considered but also the willingness of the few who are prepared to devote themselves to their community. This willingness is a remarkable advance, among many others.

The progress made

The creation of village health teams in the Maradi Department has led to considerable improvement in the standard of health in the villages, of health personnel, and of rural health organization.

The effect on the villages

In most villages, after the village health worker has been functioning for some months the number of cases of conjunctivitis decreases and wounds and skin infections heal up. In many cases there is also a marked improvement in the cleanliness of the village. The improvement in health care at the village level is such that it is very rare for a village community to refuse to develop its own scheme of village health workers.

Most often, even after temporary failure, new candidates are replacing those who abandoned their tasks. In other places it has been recorded that village health workers did not hesitate to walk dozens of kilometers to replenish their stock of drugs. Each year many villages apply for the training of village health workers, although the health services are not always able to comply with these requests because of lack of equipment and of the manpower needed for supervision.

In villages whose traditional birth attendants have received training, umbilical wounds cicatrize rapidly and although the attendants are not always called in at the beginning of labour, women experiencing difficult child birth are referred elsewhere at an earlier stage than formerly. The traditional birth attendants in villages near a dispensary accompany pregnant women and children to the clinics for expectant mothers and infants organized by the nurse and participate in health and nutrition education demonstrations.

In fact, the village health workers and traditional birth attendants in the Department of Maradi are participating directly in the education efforts being made jointly by the health services, the extension and literacy services, and the education and training services, who have selected priority educational topics and have designed for each of them flannelgraphs with figures and texts in the vernacular language (Hausa).

The first topic dealt with was weaning food, the aim of the education programme being to persuade mothers to improve the traditional pap (prepared with millet wheat not cooked in water) by cooking it after adding local products with high protein concentration (ground-nut cake, milk, or eggs). In spite of a certain resistance to these changes the new weaning pap cooked with ground-nut cake is being more and more accepted and appreciated by the mothers. The improved preparation is being demonstrated in most villages by the dispensary attendant, the village health workers, or the traditional birth attendants, or even in the centres for rural extension and literacy.

The results of the programme can be seen in the growth charts, and knowledge of nutrition, which has a direct impact on the health status of the infants, is much more widespread than knowledge of the hygiene of the body, of the pregnant women, or of the settlement.

Village health workers and traditional birth attendants have helped in the distribution of flour (provided as part of UNICEF aid to populations suffering from drought) for children under 6 years of age, giving demonstrations of how to prepare gruel.

The role of the nurses

Since the nurses have been involved in the training and inspection of village health workers and traditional birth attendants, they have been obliged themselves to learn hygiene and nutrition; they have also discovered their sector and have become educators, whereas formerly they did no more than give some treatment to patients who arrived at their dispensary. Maternal and child welfare, previously unthinkable in the absence of a female nurse, is now practised in all the rural dispensaries, although they have only one male nurse.

Formerly this nurse saw only the patients he was called in to attend but now he has less hesitation in making contact with the villagers and interesting himself in their problems, whether there are village health workers or not. This geographical and technical mobilization of the nurses appears to be one of the most important results, since it constitutes the basis for the health services development of the country.

The effect on the rural health organization

The rural health organization, until now so poor (one dispensary for every 30 000–50 000 inhabitants) and so ineffective (15% of the sick treated) has been enriched by village health teams, 7–10 of which, on an average, give as much care as one rural dispensary.

Formerly the final link in the chain, oriented more towards the town than the countryside, the dispensary is now becoming a health centre that is active all over a region. The village health workers go there for training and refresher courses, while the nurse regularly supplies, in their own villages, the necessary technical, material, and psychological support for their voluntary health activities.

Although, owing to the activities of a few village health teams, the health care activities have increased by about 20–50%, depending on the area, and many villages now receive regular monthly visits from a nurse who acts not only as healer but also as educator, the progress achieved to date is far greater than is suggested by these figures.

In fact, the training and organization of village health teams has profoundly modified the way of thinking and the behaviour not only of the health personnel and the villagers but also of the administrators and personnel in other services. All are much better informed about curative, nutritional, and preventive problems and no longer consider the health services as budget-consuming. Instead they now accept that the health services must be integrated into the programme for local and regional development.

For several years now, the responsible authorities of the Department of Maradi have been promoting a wide range of activities—maternal and child health, malaria chemoprophylaxis, health education, vaccinations, the retraining of nurses, and the extension of village health teams at the rate of 5 teams per year in each health area. Progress may, at first glance. appear to be rather slow, but the programme must take into account the availability of the technical and manpower resources required for the training and the indispensable monthly supervision. By developing steadily, the programme ensures the gradual introduction of the health service in rural areas.

The present status of the programme

Of a total of 108 village pharmacies in the Maradi Department, 20 had become completely inactive by 1 January 1974. The village health workers had given up because they were poorly motivated, not supported by the village, or too irregularly inspected (and aided) by the health personnel. After further motivation of the population and a new training course it was possible to reopen 12 pharmacies, while 29 were created during the first half of 1974, which gives, to date, a total of 129 pharmacies.

Moreover, the management committees of many village pharmacies have disappeared because of their inefficiency or embezzlement of funds by one of the members. In most of these pharmacies one of the village health workers still remaining active has then taken over the book-keeping of the drugs, which he does very well. In some cases the embezzled money, which was needed for renewing supplies of drugs to be paid for, could be recovered after discussion with the village health workers and the management committee in the presence of the villagers, who, themselves, decided what solution should be found for the problem.

All these difficulties and failures have recurred in the course of the year since the creation of the first village pharmacies and their basic cause is inadequate motivation of the population and too irregular inspection, the village health workers and the management committee having been poorly chosen or, like the other villagers, having misunderstood their role and the organization of the pharmacy.

These defects in motivation and supervision derive more from lack of awareness or extension work among the nurses themselves than from lack of resources; it is easier to wait for the patient to come to the dispensary than to help the villagers organize themselves so as to prevent and control disease. Indeed, many tours of duty for arousal or inspection have been shortened so that the nurse could return rapidly to the dispensary, whereas, with a little patience and some fatigue, three or four pharmacies could have been made to run smoothly and achieve the equivalent of 4 months' work by a dispensary.

In addition, many examples have shown that when sufficient time is taken to explain in detail to all the villagers (men and women), during several meetings if necessary, any difficulty that may arise, they are then able to assume their responsibilities and to decide on a solution suitable for the village. This has happened in cases where embezzled money has been recovered or the pharmacy run by a member of the committee or a single village health worker.

At first sight, the training of the traditional birth attendants seems to have met with fewer failures; in fact, although on 1 January 1974 there were 266 village midwives in the department, 16 were completely inactive, either because of age or infirmity (blindness) or because they were too much attached to a particular family.

Thus, the same faults, as regards motivation and inspection, are found again with, however, a few special features: on the one hand, since the traditional birth attendant always receives a present on the occasion of a birth, she is more interested in her duties than the village health worker, who is in theory entirely unrewarded; on the other hand, in order to practise, particularly if she is young (which is preferable), a traditional birth attendant must obtain the consent not only of the women but also of her husband and the other men. The motivation of the population therefore needs be carried out with great patience and thoroughness, which is not always the case.

Nevertheless, despite these difficulties the traditional birth attendants render valuable service in view of the very small number of maternity clinics. To improve maternity care, 73 new traditional birth attendants were trained in the first half of 1974 for 27 further villages, and 47 others were given refresher courses. There are now a total of 323 traditional birth attendants at work in 113 villages.

Conclusions

The village health team, comprising the traditional birth attendants and the village health workers (equipped with pharmacy kits) constitutes the basic health unit, which can provide indispensable basic medical care, maternal and child welfare, sanitation, and health education for the population of the village (and of neighbouring villages).

At the same time, the rural dispensary, which was formerly self-contained, has become a rural health centre where a regional health action plan can be worked out and where village health workers can be trained and given refresher courses, the nurse carrying on extension and educational work among the population for whom he is responsible.

To ensure the success of this health extension operation, it must be unceasingly adapted to the terrain and the circumstances so that the village health team becomes an integral part and a manifestation of the village.

Furthermore, it is necessary for health personnel at all levels (district, department, and national) periodically to review their medical activities jointly with all the services concerned, so that they can be made more general (curative, preventive, and educational) and take more account of the different geographical and socioeconomic factors at work in the country. In brief, extension work among the health personnel should help them to train and mobilize themselves to promote public health. The setting up of village health teams should be considered not as a simple technical recipe but rather as the consolidation of a public health orientation that aims at the organization of rural health services adapted to a population living in a more diversified and less well organized sphere than urban populations. For these reasons, the success and extension of these operations depend more on the mobilization (animation and motivation) of the health personnel than that of the population, who always appear to be prepared to participate in beneficial activities provided they are clearly explained from the outset. Therefore, medical officers and nurses should shift from their traditional hospital-oriented outlook to the practice of more comprehensive care in which the treatment of the individual constitutes only a step towards the definition of the geographical and socioeconomic problems of health and towards the solutions to be applied to them.

It is also obvious that the outcome of what has been achieved in the Department of Maradi, of what is going on, and what is going to develop will depend on a continuous teamwork approach at all levels and among everybody involved, the aim being to adapt the health services to the population being served. Thanks to the active participation of the people, health workers will be covering the entire populations living in remote areas, and physicians and nurses will be able fully to accomplish their task as educators, extension workers, and relievers of suffering.

MEETING BASIC HEALTH NEEDS IN TANZANIA

W. K. CHAGULA & E. TARIMO [a]

Tanzania, like many other developing countries, is committed to providing health care for everyone. This commitment has to be met within the constraints of very limited resources and inadequate data and its fulfilment has proved a formidable task in the rural areas, where the majority of the population live but which have long been neglected in comparison with urban areas. There follows a brief description of Tanzania's basic characteristics and an account of the former conditions of the health services in Tanzania, the origins of the approach that was adopted in order to improve them, the problems encountered, and the progress that has been made so far.

Tanzania's basic characteristics

General characteristics

Tanganyika is a large country (area approximately 1 million km²) situated on the east coast of Africa. It became independent in 1961 after 77 years of colonial rule. Zanzibar consists of two islands in the Indian Ocean, adjacent to Tanganyika. It became independent in 1963 after over 300 years of foreign rule. The union of Tanganyika and Zanzibar in 1964 brought the present United Republic of Tanzania into being. The following account refers only to the mainland, the former Tanganyika.

Despite its proximity to the equator, Tanzania has, by virtue of its altitude, a largely subtropical climate. Apart from the few mountains, which to the north include Kilimanjaro, the highest mountain in Africa, most of the country forms a plateau 3000–4000 feet above sea level, characterized by a combination of grassland and woodland with small areas under cultivation. It has been estimated that 75% of the land is either uninhabited or difficult to manage because of the tsetse or lack of reliable rainfall.

a In collaboration with V. Djukanović and E. Kalimo, Division of Strengthening of Health Services, World Health Organization, Geneva, Switzerland.

145

Demographic features

The last population census in 1967 revealed a total population of 12 255 000 (*1*) with a growth rate of 2.5–3% a year. Although the overall density of population is low (13 persons per km²), some areas, such as those on the lower slopes of Mount Kilimanjaro, in the coastal regions, and the southern shores of Lake Victoria, are densely populated. About 6.2% of the population lives in urban areas, the largest city, Dar es Salaam, having a population of about 500 000.

TABLE 1. ESTIMATED POPULATION OF TANZANIA
BY AGE, SEX, AND AREAS OF RESIDENCE, 1973

Age	Sex		Total	Residents in towns of more than 10 000 population	Residing in the rest of the country
	male	female			
0–4	1 250 000	1 303 000	2 553 000	149 000	2 404 000
5–14	1 840 000	1 886 000	3 726 000	154 000	3 572 000
15+	3 710 000	3 811 000	7 521 000	663 000	6 580 000
Total	6 800 000	7 000 000	13 800 000	966 000	12 834 000

Table 1 shows the main estimated population characteristics of Tanzania for 1973. The present crude death rate for Tanzania is estimated at 22 per 1000, the birth rate at about 47 per 1000, the infant mortality rate 160–165 per 1000 live births, and the expectation of life at birth 40–41 years.

The sociopolitical situation

Tanzania is administered at three levels: central, regional, and district. This applies to both Government Ministries and the only political party, the Tanganyika African National Union (TANU). With the recent adoption by the Government of a decentralization policy, the regions and districts are now able to make a wider range of decisions without reference to the central administration. The districts are divided into divisions, which are in turn divided into administrative wards. Each ward consists of "ten cell" units. Each ten cell unit comprises 10 households and is headed by an elected TANU leader, the ten cell leader.

The concept of the "Ujamaa village" has recently been receiving great emphasis throughout the country. This concept is a direct result of the Party's and the Government's attempt to provide for coordinated, organic, and purposeful development strategies at the grass roots, particularly in the rural areas. An economically viable village consists of 100–500 families working on a communal basis. It is estimated that nearly 3 million people are now living in Ujamaa villages. The target is that all the rural population will be living in Ujamaa villages by 1976.

146

Tanzania's current sociopolitical policy was set forth in the Arusha Declaration (2) promulgated by TANU in February 1967. This policy emphasizes:

(1) rural development;

(2) Government mobilization of all the country's resources for the elimination of poverty, ignorance, and disease, which were declared priority areas;

(3) local contribution (self-reliance) as an instrument for self-liberation and socioeconomic development (self-reliance was proclaimed to be of primary importance, and aid from other countries was to be used to supplement national effort; foreign aid should not be relied upon as a major instrument of development);

(4) people, land, sound policies, and good leadership as prerequisites for development; and

(5) state control and ownership of all the major means of production and distribution, and the elimination of exploitation and privileges for minorities.

Economic development

Tanzania's economic development has been slower than that of her neighbours, partly owing to the political uncertainties associated with the system of mandates and trusteeships under which the country was governed before it became independent. Under these systems the colonial authorities could not be assured of their future and permanent status in Tanganyika as was the case in their other colonies. In terms of annual *per capita* income (approximately $100) Tanzania is one of the 25 least developed of the developing countries in the world. According to King (3), it is impossible to provide basic health services "on any but the most minimal scale when the annual *per capita* income is less than about £25". This is obviously a serious stumbling-block to the Government's efforts at improving basic health services in the rural areas. The goals of several previous health plans were not realized, mainly because the economic realities of the country were not properly taken into consideration.

Education policy

Tanzania's broad objectives for education are the attainment of self-reliance in high-level and middle-level manpower by 1980 and adult literacy by 1975. The general education policy of the country took a new turn in 1967 with the adoption of a policy of "education for self-reliance" (4). Under this policy, primary and secondary education was no longer to be

147

regarded as a stepping-stone to higher education, but rather as a means to enable people to serve the Nation and to contribute as effectively as possible to development. At present only about 50% of school-age children attend primary school, which is free to all children who can gain admission. This represents an increase of approximately 70% between 1961 and 1971.

Major health problems

The major causes of morbidity and mortality in Tanzania, as in most developing countries, are infectious and parasitic diseases. Two other problem areas are defective nutrition and maternal morbidity and mortality. In all, poverty-linked diseases account for about three-quarters of all deaths, while the diseases common in affluent countries, such as heart diseases, are relatively unimportant. Malaria is the leading cause of hospital attendance and admissions. Table 2 gives the leading causes of mortality

TABLE 2. COMMONEST CAUSES OF DEATH IN HOSPITAL IN TANZANIA, 1972

Disease	Percentage of total deaths (51 000)
Pneumonia (all forms)	15.6
Measles	10.5
Gastroenteritis (all forms)	9.6
Conditions of early infancy	6.9
Defective nutrition	5.1
Tuberculosis (all forms)	4.7
Tetanus	4.6
Heart disease	4.5
Malaria	4.4
Anaemia (all forms)	3.8

in Tanzania. The data must, however, be interpreted with caution as the country's statistical systems are still in a rudimentary state; for instance, there is at present no compulsory registration of births and deaths in most parts of the country.

The original health situation

The country's first government medical department was set up by the German colonial government in 1891 to safeguard the health of government employees. This service was disrupted during the First World War, and it was not until 1923 that Britain, to whom the mandate for administering Tanganyika was assigned by the League of Nations, was able to re-establish a similar medical service. Since then, several attempts have been made to plan the further development of the country's health services. There have been four major reports on this topic, three of which were

148

formulated before Tanzania became independent in 1961. The 1947 post-war development plan (5) was very ambitious, envisaging, for instance, that over the following 20 years 2000 doctors and 40 000 hospital beds would become available—now, 27 years later, only 500 doctors and 18 000 beds are available. In 1949, Dr. E. Pridie, then the Chief Medical Adviser to the British Colonial Office, also undertook a review of health service policy in Tanganyika (6). Another review was undertaken by the colonial government's Medical Department in 1956, and a 5-year development plan was prepared (7). Like the 1949 report, this review recommended that emphasis in the provision of health services should be placed on the development of rural health centres. Titmuss observed in 1964 that none of the previous three plans had achieved its stated objectives (8); he also stressed the need for more rural health centres. Despite these reports, not much impact was made in terms of the development of health services in the rural areas, which can roughly be measured by the number of new dispensaries and rural health centres, particularly the latter.

Health centres

As far back as 1938, the creation of health centres was being advocated: "The dispensary must become a health centre" (9). It was not, however, until the early 1950s that the first one was established. In the 5-year development plan drawn up in 1956, the Medical Department emphasized the need for health centres and proposed that, of the estimated total require-

TABLE 3.   THE DEVELOPMENT OF HEALTH FACILITIES IN TANZANIA

	1961	1965	1969	1971	1973	1980 [a]
Rural health centres	22	40	50	87	108	300
Dispensaries	975	1236	1362	1436	1515	2200
Hospitals	98	109	121	123	123	130
Outpatient visits per person	1.9	3.0	3.4	4.0	5.0	
Admissions per 1000 people	29.7	34.8	39.0	42.6	64.5	

[a] Projections.

ment of 160 rural health centres (to give a ratio of one centre to every 50 000 people), 40 should be built during the period 1956–1961. Table 3 shows that only 22 rural health centres were in operation by the end of 1961, and at the end of 1965 their number had only slightly increased to 40.

Dispensaries

The rate of development of dispensaries has been slightly better, as Table 3 shows. Until recently, when village health posts were introduced, these units were the smallest. Dispensaries and rural health centres were administered by local authorities until the abolition of these authorities in 1972, when the centres were taken over by the Ministry of Health. The development of these units had therefore largely depended on the financial capacity as well as the competence and interest in health matters of the various local authorities.

Hospitals

In Tanzania, the district hospital and the various health centres and dispensaries in a district constitute the basic health units. It is held that support and supervision from district hospitals is essential if dispensaries and rural health centres are to be really useful. This is why in Tanzania a discussion of basic health units is considered incomplete unless hospitals are mentioned. Table 3 shows that the development of hospitals in the last 5 years has been much slower than that of other health service facilities.

Distribution of health service centres

As in some other developing countries, not only have the basic health service centres been generally inadequate to meet the needs of the people but they have also tended to be concentrated in a few areas. In Tanzania, the colonial governments generally built hospitals in the large towns, and this trend was followed in the first few years of independence. Missionary health centres tended to be located in densely populated rural areas but have been much more active in some regions than others. These are the two main reasons for the inadequate distribution of health service centres in the country.

The ratios of doctors or beds to population are often used to measure quantitative adequacy. At the end of 1967, the doctor/population ratio was 1:24 000, but this ratio varied greatly in the various administrative districts, and the number of doctors has not increased much in recent years. The hospital bed/population ratio ranged between 1:400 and 1:3500 in the various districts, with a national average of 1:800. There were 1236 dispensaries in the country in 1965, giving a dispensary/population ratio of 1:9500, with great variation from district to district. The ratio of rural health centres to population also varied greatly from district to district.

Another measure of the adequacy of health services is that of expenditure per head in the various districts. There have always been considerable differences in the annual *per capita* expenditure on health services in the various districts; the present range is from TSh 2 to TSh 90.

A special study of the geographical distribution of health service centres has recently been carried out by the University of Dar es Salaam in close collaboration with the Ministry of Health. The distribution of the population (as shown by the 1967 census) was superimposed on a map of Tanzania showing the location of hospitals, rural health centres, and dispensaries. A distance of 10 km was chosen for the purposes of the study, on the assumption that most villagers would be prepared to walk for about two hours to obtain treatment for ordinary complaints at a health service centre. The study showed that some 2½ million people, or about 10% of the population, live more than 10 km from any health service centre; this percentage varied from 2% to 40% in the different districts. It was also found that only about 25% of the population lived within 10 km of a hospital.

Another measure of the degree of access to health care is the way in which the health services are used by people in the various parts of the country. As medical care in Tanzania is, generally speaking, free of charge, hospital charges do not constitute a barrier to access to health services. This does not, however, mean a complete absence of economic barriers; economic factors may often determine whether a patient comes to hospital or not—for instance, bus or railway fares can be beyond the means of the average peasant. The urban population in 1967 (6.2% of the total population—see Table 1) accounted for over 25% of all admissions to government hospitals and more than half of the outpatient consultations.

The origins of the present approach

The above considerations make it obvious that a change in approach was absolutely necessary if any degree of equitable distribution of health care was to be achieved. Reference has already been made to the 1967 Arusha Declaration by TANU (2), which laid down Tanzania's social and economic policy.

We must not forget that people who live in towns can possibly become exploiters of those who live in rural areas. All our big hospitals are in towns and they benefit only a small section of the people of Tanzania; it is the overseas sale of the peasants' produce which provides the foreign exchange of payment. Those who do not get the benefit of the hospitals thus carry the major responsibility for paying for them.

The Arusha Declaration directed that rural areas should receive priority in development programmes. Poverty, ignorance, and disease were declared priority areas. The same problems had already been declared priority areas by TANU when it was founded in 1954, so that it is probably more appropriate to refer to the Constitution of TANU (10) as the origin of the approach.

At the 1971 TANU Biennial Conference, the need for increased rural development was re-emphasized. TANU directed, in particular, that health services, adequate and wholesome water, and education for the people, particularly in the rural areas, should receive priority in all the country's future annual development plans. Since these declarations, many leaders, including the President himself, have frequently spent long periods in rural areas helping in the implementation of various development projects. On the whole, considerable development has taken place in the rural areas. The Ministry of Health has had to translate this and other Party directives into action. The present approach towards meeting the basic health needs of the country can therefore be traced to the Party, which has directed the Government.

The approach and methods adopted

The present approach is mainly based on a realization that, with limited resources and unlimited problems, priorities have to be worked out carefully. President Nyerere, introducing the Second Five-Year Development Plan at the 1969 TANU Biennial Conference, said, "To plan is to choose". His words, which are repeated in all corners of the country, are a constant reminder of this need.

Emphasis on disease prevention

The Government places great emphasis on disease prevention programmes. This policy has a long history, but its implementation has not been easy. For example, it was stated explicitly in the Second Five-Year Development Plan: "The 1969–74 Health Plan is directed above all towards the development of preventive and rural health services in a positive and dynamic manner". An analysis of the results of this and other plans shows that, in general, achievements in preventive programmes have been minimal. It is only in the field of maternal and child health and smallpox control that there has been considerable success. In an attempt to rectify the situation, the government has taken or is considering remedial measures. For instance, the Ministry of Health has been reorganized and a Directorate of Preventive Services has been established to deal with the development of disease prevention programmes. Other possible remedial measures under consideration include setting aside a certain percentage of the annual health budget for disease prevention programmes.

However, the contrasting of the curative with the preventive concept is of limited value in Tanzania, where the aim is to provide a comprehensive health service for all. In the first place, it is not easy to define the activities that should fall under disease prevention programmes. For example, in a number of countries, dispensaries, rural health centres, public health laboratories, and schools for the training of public health workers form part of the preventive services. Secondly, a health service infrastructure is essential if lasting success is to be achieved in preventive health campaigns and health promotion activities. Thus, although in Tanzania dispensaries and rural health centres are not directly the responsibility of the Preventive Service Directorate, their development on the lines to be discussed later is essential for effective disease prevention. The discussion on these health service centres will highlight the fact that they all provide both curative and preventive health services. This combined approach is also essential in the control of many diseases, particularly communicable diseases, where the treatment of cases must be combined with preventive measures.

Community involvement

In Tanzania, community involvement in projects starts at the planning stage. The Party and the Government emphasize the need to involve the people in the planning of projects—the aim is to develop people's projects rather than impose projects on the people. Thus, the TANU Guidelines of 1971 state: "The duty of our Party is not to urge the people to implement plans which have been decided upon by a few experts and leaders. The duty of our Party is to ensure that the leaders and experts implement the plans that have been agreed upon by the people themselves" (11). One of the aims of the recent decentralization of government was to allow for more community involvement, not only in the planning of projects and programmes but also in their implementation. At each administrative level—village, district, region, and national headquarters—there are planning committees consisting of both technocrats and elected representatives of the people. Centrally, the Ministry of Economic Affairs and Development Planning, in collaboration with the Office of the Prime Minister, is responsible for giving broad guidelines regarding priorities and national strategies.

Many health projects are being implemented by Tanzanians through various nation-building activities. These include the construction of dispensaries, rural health centres, and extensions to hospital wards. Most development projects in Tanzania include an element of self-help. Thus, in the construction of a health centre, certain buildings such as kitchens and mortuaries are not usually provided for in the financial estimates; it is expected that they will be built on a self-help basis. In this way, the urge to help in nation-building is directed to the right areas. All national building projects (that are not supplementary to government projects) have to be approved by the appropriate local development committees in the same way as any other projects.

Nation-building activities are not limited to development projects. The recent campaign to keep many Tanzanian towns clean is a good example of other types of self-help. Nation-building activities are also a feature of projects that come under the auspices of other government ministries but have a direct effect on the health of the people. Thus, the Ntomoko project, in which 124 km of water trench was dug on a self-help basis, will greatly improve the health of the people in the 23 villages to be served by the water pipe-line. The role of self-help in Tanzania is an extremely important one; in the last few years the impetus for improved environmental health services in the rural areas has probably been developed not so much by the Ministry of Health as through government-encouraged community self-help schemes.

This involvement of the people has at least three advantages. First, it facilitates better coordination of development projects. Secondly, people are more likely to be willing to participate in the implementation of projects that they have helped to plan. Thus, since the decentralization of government many more health development projects such as dispensaries and rural health centres have been completed each year than before. Thirdly, the element of self-help in the implementation of projects is encouraged.

The role of Ujamaa villages

As was mentioned above, nearly 3 million Tanzanians are now living and working communally in Ujamaa villages and it is expected that by the end of 1976 the whole of Tanzania's rural population will be living in these villages.

TANU's decision to mobilize Tanzania's rural population into Ujamaa villages has two main objectives: the first is to make it easier for the government to provide the people with facilities such as adequate and wholesome water, education, and basic health services; the second is to raise productivity so that the villages can more effectively combat the vicious circle of poverty, ignorance, and disease, which were the original enemies of TANU when the Party was fighting for political independence. Thus, the Tanzanian Ujamaa village policy indirectly contributes to the general betterment of the health of the rural population; the importance of these villages as bases for disease prevention campaigns and health education programmes will be mentioned later.

The role of rural development workers

The development of health services is incorporated into overall rural development. For the training of rural development workers, both men and women, several institutions have been established. The courses aim at widening the horizon and understanding of the rural development workers in the various aspects of development, which is pregnant with economic, political, social, and psychological implications. The courses are primarily intended for the front-line rural development workers who are to live and work hand-in-hand with the villagers in implementing the national development plans the Ujamaa way. Thus it is necessary that this basic training in rural development should emphasize practical rural skills in their totality. To this end, rural development workers stimulate communities to recognize their main health problems and motivate them to see the need to take action towards eradicating these problems. They also help communities to choose the best remedial measures and assist them to implement measures chosen.

Mass health education

The campaign popularly known as *"Mtu ni Afya"*, or *"Man is Health"*, is a good example of the effective use currently being made of other Government Ministries and organizations to increase the effectiveness of the health budget. The project was planned in close collaboration with the Adult Education Directorate of the Ministry of National Education, who were anxious to ensure that literate villagers were continually supplied with reading material so that they would not relapse into illiteracy. Besides providing reading material, the project aimed at giving villagers information on the symptoms and prevention of common diseases. The materials for the project were prepared by the Health Education Unit of the Ministry of Health. The painstaking preparatory phase included seminars for "teachers" at regional, district, and divisional levels.

The project was formally launched in April 1973, with some 75 000 study groups, and a total population of 2 million took part. Radio broadcasts, including two speeches by the Prime Minister, and the wide distribution of magazines, newspapers, booklets, and posters were used to disseminate the health information. This group approach of the campaign increased the participants' awareness and encouraged group action to bring about better health for the group. Discussions were held after the groups had listened to a radio programme or read a relevant section in a magazine.

The cost of the campaign was very low—TSh 1.40 (US$0.20) per participant. The campaign is one in a series of mass adult education efforts, and several independent evaluations indicate that it was one of Tanzania's most successful campaigns. Others are now being planned on similar lines. The next one, to be known as *"Chakula ni Uhai"*, or *"Food is Life"*, will be launched soon. It will probably be followed by another on environmental sanitation.

Health service facilities in the rural areas of Tanzania

The type of health service facility provided is largely determined by the size of the population it is to serve.

The overall objective of the present health care programme in Tanzania is to achieve a better coverage of the population. The capital cost of a dispensary is about TSh 52 000 and the cost of running it is about

TSh 30 000 per year [a]   The corresponding figures for a health centre are TSh 600 000 and 150 000 respectively. A hospital bed costs about TSh 25 000–140 000 to provide and TSh 30–60 per day to operate. It is therefore obvious that the highest priority in the development budget should be given to the extension of rural health centres and dispensaries if Tanzania's limited resources are to be as effectively utilized as possible. Moreover, the training of the necessary staff must be coordinated with the construction of the health service centres. The average costs of training a doctor, medical assistant, and rural medical aide are approximately TSh 250 000, 15 000, and 10 000 respectively. Emphasis therefore needs to be placed on the training of primary health workers.

Village health posts

There is usually only one village health post for each Ujamaa village. This is the smallest centre, which provides treatment for minor ailments and also offers first-aid treatment for more serious illness and injury. But, probably even more important, the centre provides the village with a base for health campaigns. In the case of village health posts, buildings play a relatively minor role, and, therefore, simple structures or existing buildings, such as part of a school or primary cooperative society, are normally used in the delivery of these services. Such centres are mostly meant for Ujamaa villages in their initial stages of development, for as the villages grow in size, the centres are usually upgraded to dispensaries.

Rural Dispensaries

There are now 1555 dispensaries in the country (300 run by voluntary agencies), giving a dispensary/population ratio of 1:9000. The main criterion used in the allocation of rural dispensaries is the size of the population to be served by a dispensary. The target is that by 1980 there should be one dispensary for every 6000–8000 people. To meet this target, 100 dispensaries are being built every year, priority being given to areas with the worst ratios. Other factors considered when dispensaries are being allocated include the percentage of population living in Ujamaa villages and the general accessibility of the various parts of an administrative district.

A standard design for a dispensary unit has been prepared. The key building is the dispensary block, providing rooms for waiting, examinations, dressings, medicines, laboratory, and injections. The unit also has a latrine block, and staff quarters. Although it may also have two blocks for holding beds and another two for maternity cases, its main function is to provide outpatient treatment and serve as a centre for the organizing and running of health campaigns. A dispensary is generally staffed by

---

[a] TSh. 7.14 = US$1.00 (1974).

a rural medical aide (in charge), a maternal and child health aide, a health auxiliary, and one or two supporting staff.

Rural health centres

There are now (1974) 108 rural health centres functioning in the country, giving a centre/population ratio of 1:99 750. In order to reach the target ratio of 1:50 000 by 1980, 25 centres are being constructed annually. Other factors also being taken into consideration in the allocation of rural health centres include the accessibility of existing rural health centres, the accessibility of district hospitals, and the proviso that no administrative district should have, at present, more than 6 rural health centres.

A standard design for a rural health centre has been prepared. Besides the dispensary, the rural health centre has a total of 14 beds—6 maternity and 8 holding. These units are manned by 7–9 medical auxiliaries, including a medical assistant (in charge), a nurse, 2 rural medical aides, and a health auxiliary. The centres provide both curative and preventive medical care, with emphasis on the latter. Each centre supervises the dispensaries in its catchment area, usually 4 or 5 in number. The centre also provides a mobile health service for remote parts of its catchment area.

Hospitals

There are 123 hospitals (60 run by voluntary agencies) in the country with a total of about 18 000 beds (8000 belonging to voluntary agencies). The following factors are taken into account when hospital beds are being allocated:

(*a*) the total increase in hospital beds—this should be 3% (i.e., about 300 beds for the whole country) per annum to cater for the increase in population;

(*b*) the number of beds per district—each district should have a hospital of about 60–100 beds;

(*c*) the average bed/population ratio in the various districts—the 1980 target for beds in government-operated hospitals is 1:1000;

(*d*) the utilization of existing hospital beds;

(*e*) the existing or proposed training schemes at each hospital; and

(*f*) the accessibility of the hospitals.

District hospitals are under the supervision of regional hospitals. Cases from district hospitals are referred to regional and consultant hospitals (there are 3 consultant hospitals at present). The expansion of hospitals is not currently a priority area. The only hospital development continuously undertaken is the improvement of the ancillary facilities, (e.g., laundry, kitchen, theatre, and stores) and the provision of additional staff quarters, in order to improve the quality of the services provided.

Mobile health services

Mobile health services are based in rural health centres and hospitals. The mobile health service teams provide both curative and preventive services to people in the remote rural areas. These preventive services include health education, communicable disease control, the improvement of environmental sanitation, and maternal and child health clinics.

Health service manpower for rural areas

Medical auxiliaries or primary health workers are easier to recruit and much cheaper to train and employ than physicians. They also work more effectively in rural areas than those with university education (*12*). As mentioned above, only 25% of the population of Tanzania live within 10 km of a hospital whereas 90% live within 10 km of a rural health centre or a dispensary. This means that some 65% of the population receive care from primary health workers, who fulfil the function of general medical practitioners and are the mainstay of Tanzania's rural health services. The more important primary health workers in Tanzania are described below. The training and development of health services manpower is the direct responsibility of the Ministry of Health and is not a decentralized function.

Village medical helpers

Village medical helpers are selected by fellow villagers, when they leave primary school after 7 years of education, to undergo 3–6 months' training at a district hospital. Their training enables them (1) to treat minor ailments, (2) to provide first-aid treatment for the more serious diseases, and (3) to help villagers in the prevention of common diseases.

Maternal and child health aides

The functions of maternal and child health aides (MCH aides) are:

(*a*) to organize and run maternal health services, including the provision of antenatal and postnatal care, and to recognize at-risk patients;

(*b*) to conduct normal deliveries;

(*c*) to organize and conduct clinics for preschool children (under-fives);

(*d*) to provide health education; and

(*e*) to participate in family and school health activities.

MCH aides are intended to form the base of a pyramid of skills in public health nursing, community nursing, and midwifery and will work primarily in dispensaries and rural health centres, the target being to have at least one MCH aide at each of these establishments.

158

In all, 19 schools for MCH aides, one in each administrative region, are to be built in 1974 and 1975 with bilateral assistance, and will supersede the 10 existing schools that are training village midwives. At present these schools do not have a uniform curriculum, the duration of their courses varying from 6 months to 2 years. The MCH aide will be an improvement on the village midwife in three ways. First, the MCH aide will be trained according to a standardized national curriculum lasting 18 months, including 6 months of practical field training; the minimum basic requirement for admission into the course remains primary education. Secondly, family planning, not at present taught to village midwives, will be introduced into the training of the MCH aides, who should at least be able to continue providing family planning services initiated at a higher level. Thirdly, nutrition education at the village level will be emphasized in the curriculum for MCH aides.

Health auxiliaries

Health auxiliaries have been trained and employed in environmental sanitation work in rural areas over the past 8 years. Their training curriculum is currently being revised, but the basic admission requirement of at least a primary school leaving certificate will remain, and preference will continue to be given to those with previous experience in the fields of health and community development. Health auxiliaries are employed at both rural health centres and dispensaries. Their functions include:

(*a*) the provision of general health education;

(*b*) the promotion of village sanitation through health education, visits to homes, schools, communal centres, and participation in activities considered necessary to improve environmental health;

(*c*) getting to know the community in which they work, so as to be in a position to assist in tracing outpatients who default or fail to attend regularly for treatment; and

(*d*) participation in campaigns conducted against specific diseases.

At present there are three health auxiliary schools, and more are expected to be built before 1980.

Rural medical aides

A rural medical aide has received at least primary school education and undergoes a medical training course lasting at least 3 years. His main functions include:

(*a*) outpatient treatment of simple diseases;

159

(*b*) initial treatment of serious illness, pending referral to a rural health centre or hospital;

(*c*) aftercare, if required, of patients discharged from hospital; and

(*d*) participation in immunization and community health programmes.

There are currently 10 schools for rural medical aides. The target is to have 16 schools by 1980, when there should be 2800 rural medical aides to man the 2200 dispensaries and 300 health centres expected to be available. The aim of the rural medical aide's training programme is to produce a physician's substitute—he is the doctor at the dispensary and the rural health centre and not necessarily a physician's helper. The rural medical aide's curriculum is currently being revised. He will gradually replace the present dispensary assistants (formerly known as tribal dressers), who were developed in the mid-1920s to man the local authority dispensaries started at that time. Tribal dressers were selected by the chief from among the more able members of the tribe and underwent a 3-month training course in the local hospital. At the end of the course they were given an instruction pamphlet for reference, printed in English and Kiswahili. In recent years, although their selection has been made by local authorities, their training has remained casual. With an increase in the number of schools, candidates with better education became available, and so the rural medical aide course was started. A number of dispensaries still remain under the charge of tribal dressers but no more will be appointed.

Medical assistants

The most important rural health service facility in Tanzania is the rural health centre. Since the medical assistant is trained to be in charge of this type of centre, he is obviously a key person among Tanzanian rural health personnel.

Medical assistants were formerly known as "dispensers". Their training was started in the mid-1920s and consisted of a full-time 18-month course. In 1936, the course was extended to 3 years and candidates were required to have received 10 years of education. This requirement continued until 1962, when the course was abolished. The extension of secondary school education to class XII led to a reduction in class X leavers and there was also a feeling that medical assistants were not sufficiently equipped to take charge of rural health centres, which were increasingly receiving greater emphasis. The course was therefore restarted in 1968, the requirement being secondary education (7 years of primary and 4 years of secondary education).

There are at present 5 schools for medical assistants, and 2 more are planned. One provides a 2-year course for selected rural medical aides. The target is to train 1500 medical assistants by 1980.

160

Licensed medical practitioners (assistant medical officers)

Assistant medical officers can perform functions intermediate between those of a medical assistant and those of a fully qualified physician. They are medical assistants with at least 4 years of work experience who have successfully completed an 18-month up-grading course.

The course was first started in 1961. It covers general medicine, surgery, and (subjects not normally covered in a medical assistant's course) obstetrics and gynaecology. When the course was started, great controversy was aroused in the medical profession and in other circles by the decision that after their training the graduates should be licensed medical practitioners and referred to as "doctors". Some physicians felt that this title should be reserved for fully medically qualified people. On the other hand, the World Health Organization's definitions of a professional worker as "a health worker trained to the generally accepted level for that discipline in a particular country" and an auxiliary worker as "a technical worker in a particular field with less than full professional qualifications" (13) have been seriously questioned in Tanzania. "Medical auxiliaries are altogether a different type of medical personnel and are very much professionals in their own right" (14). Even the title "doctor" is now considered by some to be misleading and unfortunate in view of the various persons who share this role (15). Meanwhile, as the debate continues, the average villager continues to benefit. Often the assistant medical officer, the medical assistant, or the rural medical aide is the only "doctor" he knows.

It is not possible to describe all the types of personnel that in one way or another help in the provision of rural health services in Tanzania. It will probably suffice to mention that manpower forecasts have already been made for the following personnel: nurses, dental assistants, dental technicians, pharmaceutical assistants, dispensing auxiliaries, radiographers, radiography assistants, laboratory assistants, laboratory auxiliaries, health education officers, and physiotherapists.

There are just over 500 doctors in Tanzania, giving a doctor/population ratio of 1:23 000. As Table 4 shows, the total number of doctors in the country has not greatly changed in recent years. The target for 1980

TABLE 4. HEALTH MANPOWER DEVELOPMENT IN TANZANIA

Year	1961	1969	1971	1973	1980 a
MCH aides/village midwives	400	545	650	750	2 500
Health auxiliaries	150	180	230	325	800
Nurse/midwife " A "	388	683	838	934	1 960
Nurse/midwife " B "	984	1 619	2 110	2 690	4 100
Rural medical aides	380	462	544	621	2 800
Medical assistants	200	249	289	335	1 200
Assistant medical officers	32	103	115	140	300
Doctors: Tanzanian	12	90	155	231	700
foreign	413	355	324	302	130
Total	2 959	4 286	5 280	6 328	14 490

a Targets.

161

is 700 Tanzanian doctors and 130 foreign doctors. According to WHO's target ratio of 1:10 000, Tanzania needs 1200 doctors for her population. It is therefore obvious that reliance will continue to be placed on primary health workers or medical auxiliaries for a very long time to come.

There is still a great need to increase the production of primary health workers, but an important lesson learnt from past mistakes is that their career prospects need to be worked out more carefully. Happily, this has now been done for most types of primary health workers. Thus, the way is now open for a rural medical aide to rise to become a fully qualified medical specialist by undergoing appropriate, officially accepted up-grading courses.

Doctors

The doctor undergoes 6 years of secondary education, followed by a 5-year university course and one year of internship. The philosophy followed in the training of doctors in Tanzania is that the doctor should be educated to meet local needs and problems. Thus, at the University of Dar es Salaam, community medicine is taught throughout the 200-week course of study, and the student must spend a total of at least 11 weeks doing field work in communities. New graduates are under contract to the Government for 5 years and can be posted to any part of the country.

As mentioned earlier, there are 500 doctors in the country, excluding assistant medical officers, and the target for 1980 is 700. The postgraduate programme envisages the training of a total of 180 specialists out of the 700 doctors. These specialists will staff the faculty of medicine, the consultant hospitals, and the regional hospitals. Each administrative region will have at least 4 specialists—a surgeon, a physician, an obstetrician and gynaecologist, and a public health specialist, who will be the Regional Medical Officer.

Private medical practitioners

The role of private medical practitioners has decreased greatly in recent years. In 1968, there were 141 private practitioners out of a total of 360 physicians. The corresponding figures at the end of 1973 were 73 and 540 respectively. The private practitioners are mostly foreigners, there being very few Tanzanians in private medical practice.

Traditional medical practitioners

A significant number of Tanzanians, especially those who live far from the organized health services, continue to depend on medical care provided by traditional practioners and midwives. These indigenous systems of medicine are not yet integrated into the organized health services. There is no registration of traditional practitioners and the only requirements demanded of practitioners over the years have been: they must have a *bona fide* practice, the practitioner must be recognized by the community

162

to which he belongs as being fully trained for such practice, the practice must be among the community to which he belongs and the practice must not be dangerous.

The Government has recently decided to promote research into traditional medical care systems and the Faculty of Medicine of the University of Dar es Salaam has been called upon to cooperate with the Ministry of Health in this connexion. Bilateral aid from a country with considerable experience of research in this field and in the coordination of these systems with the organized health services is also expected soon.

Health expenditure

As the new Tanzanian health policy has only recently been implemented, most of the increase in central government health expenditure has occurred in the last 3 years. The absolute amount is still relatively low—about TSh 18 per head in 1973. In addition, the average private sector expenditure on health is about TSh 3 per head and the total health expenditure thus rises to TSh 21 per head. This shows that the country spends about 3% of its gross national product on health services, excluding water supply, sanitation, nutrition, and some other indirect but important determinants of health.

Each year TANU and the Government allocate a reasonable proportion of the total national budget for health services, commensurate with the total available national resources and in accordance with the national development priorities.

TABLE 5. HEALTH DEVELOPMENT BUDGET ESTIMATES IN TANZANIA
(EXPRESSED AS PERCENTAGES)

	1970–71	1971–72	1972–73	1973–74	1974–75
Hospital services	52 [a]	52 [b]	27 [c]	15	12
Rural health centres and dispensaries	24	33	35	33	24
Preventive services	1	2	10	2	8
Training	24 [d]	13	18 [e]	48[c]	55
Manufacturing	6	—	10	2	1

[a] About 70% in the capital city.
[b] About 60% in the capital city.
[c] Less than 10% in the capital city.
[d] Virtually all for the capital city.
[e] No expenditure for the capital city.

The implementation of the new health policy is reflected in Table 5, which shows the health development budget estimates for the last 5 years. Within the health services sector proper, the priority areas have been the construction of rural health centres and dispensaries and schools for training the various new types of health personnel. This has led to a great increase in the proportion of health resources allocated to the training of personnel, which accounts for more than half the health development budget for 1974–75. A change in the allocation of resources within the health sectors is evident from the fact that 70% of the 1972–73 national budget for health services was devoted to rural health services compared with less than 50% in the previous year.

The same trends can also be seen in government health recurrent expenditure (Table 6). Gradually, less recurrent expenditure is being devoted to

TABLE 6. TOTAL GOVERNMENT (NATIONAL AND REGIONAL) HEALTH RECURRENT EXPENDITURE IN TANZANIA (EXPRESSED AS PERCENTAGES)

	1970–71	1971–72	1972–73	1973–74	1974–75
Hospital services	79.8	78.9	71.6	69.0	60.2
Rural health centres and dispensaries	9.1	10.9	18.3	19.3	19.1
Preventive services	5.0	3.9	3.9	4.7	12.4
Training	2.4	3.1	3.5	4.8	6.3
Manufacturing	1.3	1.8	1.5	1.6	1.1
Administration	2.4	1.4	1.2	0.6	0.9

hospital services and more to rural health centres and dispensaries, preventive services, and training. As in other parts of the world, more than half the health recurrent expenditure is still being devoted to hospital services.

If the ambitious programme of rural health centres and dispensaries referred to above is to be implemented, the rapid annual increase in hospital costs must be stemmed. A decision has already been made on controlling the increase in hospital beds. Although the appropriateness of "Say's Law" (16) (supply creates its own demand) in hospitals has been questioned, the answer to the problem of overcrowding in hospitals is not necessarily an increase in the number of beds. The Ministry of Health is currently trying to work out a formula by which health service centres of a similar category can be allocated a fixed sum of money for the operation of each service, e.g., per bed, per outpatient, etc. The Ministry is also exploring ways of controlling the use of drugs, which in recent years have been consuming a disproportionate amount of the total annual budget for the health service. The aim is to lower still further the cost of providing basic health services to the majority of the people, particulary in the rural areas.

Utilization of all available resources

In addition to the government health services, the health service system in Tanzania includes the services and facilities provided by voluntary agencies, occupational health services, private practitioners, the Family Planning Association, the Flying Doctor Service, external aid, the services provided by other government ministries, and self-help. Every attempt is being made to coordinate all these facilities. In practice, this often means having a representative of the Ministry of Health on the executive boards of the various organizations. Thus, there is a senior official of the Ministry of Health on the executive boards of the Flying Doctor Service, the Dar es Salaam Group Occupational Health Service, and the Family Planning Association. The Government's priorities and policies are also disseminated to these bodies through publications and regular meetings.

Voluntary agencies

About 20 separate voluntary agencies provide health services in Tanzania. In the past, any voluntary agency could build a dispensary or health centre in any area it chose. This is no longer possible, since prior approval of the various development committees must now be obtained. In this way, duplication is avoided and health service centres are located in areas where they are most needed. Although individual hospitals or dispensaries are supervised by their own organizations, the district medical officer is increasingly assuming the role of coordinator of all the health services in his district.

Since the 1920s, the work of voluntary agencies in providing health services has been assisted by various kinds of government grant. These grants are intended to subsidize hospital charges, and in districts with no government hospital the grant to one of the voluntary agency hospitals covers all charges, so that treatment is offered free to the public. Such a hospital is referred to as a " designated district hospital ".

External health assistance

The *"Mtu ni Afya"* campaign is one of the projects that are being supported by foreign aid. In Tanzania, bilateral and multilateral aid greatly increase the effectiveness of the annual health budget. Thus, over 70% of the health development section of the 1973–74 budget was derived from these sources. It is gratifying to note that the providers of aid have tailored their assistance to the Government's priorities. Thus, the construction of dispensaries, rural health centres, and schools for medical auxiliaries is being undertaken mainly with foreign aid. Nevertheless self-reliance is proclaimed to be of primary importance and aid from other countries is not to be the major instrument of development. Hence the slogan: "Cooperation with other countries, but not with poisoned aid".

Conclusions

The health problems of Tanzania, as those of most developing countries, are enormous. What has been briefly discussed here are the ways in which Tanzania is trying to diagnose and solve these immense problems.

Tanzania's approach—solving her health problems by increasing coverage to the rural areas where a great majority of the people live—has a solid foundation in the Arusha Declaration of 1967, which is a sociopolitical statement of intent with a well-defined rural development component.

The present policy of providing clean water, universal free primary education, and health services as priorities aims at improving life in the countryside as a whole. Thus, health is seen as an integral part of an overall rural development policy.

The formulation of such a broad policy calls for the setting up of a comprehensive mechanism for planning and implementing programmes in accordance with defined priorities. In Tanzania, health services are planned at various levels and are then coordinated with the overall national development plan. This plan aims at providing services capable of meeting basic health needs of the majority of the population. Reorganization of the countryside by regrouping the population in larger villages reduces the planners' nightmare of having to plan for sparsely populated and often inaccessible areas, and further reduces the cost of providing social amenities.

Tanzania is one of the 25 countries with the lowest gross national product in the world; consequently, resources are small. By actively involving the community in health and other programmes, the authorities have been able to maximize the effect of these meagre resources. Mass mobilization is used as a deliberate political tool to raise the social consciousness of health as the people's responsibility. Specially trained development workers with orientation in health improvement help to channel the health aspirations of the community into overall development.

Tanzania's rural health units consist mainly of rural health centres and dispensaries. They are designed to provide comprehensive health services for the rural community, with special emphasis on preventive activities, although at the moment greater attention is being paid to curative medicine—to the detriment of preventive activities. However, the authorities have taken note of this fact and hope to effect a change by striking an equitable balance between curative and preventive measures.

Health manpower for the delivery of this rural health care consists of four main categories of workers: medical assistants, rural medical aides, maternal and child health aides, and health auxiliaries. These primary health workers are not substitutes for doctors. They form an integral part of a health system providing valuable service to the rural population under the supervision and with the support of the next tier of the health service.

Tanzania's approach aims at increasing the coverage and utilization of primary health services in rural areas rather than at providing sophisticated but less accessible and often expensive services. The target is that by 1980 every individual should be able to obtain at least a minimum level of care at his own village and be referred to a somewhat higher level of care, a few kilometres away, so that there will be wider coverage and a more equitable distribution of services in accordance with the stated objectives. The use of primary health workers maximizes the use of resources at minimal cost to give wider coverage.

166

However, in spite of the many innovative features in Tanzania's approach, the health situation in 1974 in terms of meeting the basic needs of the whole population is still inadequate. The reasons for this inadequacy are varied; among them are the historical past and the fact that the Tanzanian government had to start almost from scratch. The major constraint has been economic and the lack of suitably trained manpower. Within the last three years, as a consequence of changed national priorities and the allocation of more funds to rural health services, efforts have been made to build more rural health centres and dispensaries; many schools for training rural health workers have also been built, so that the majority of the population can be covered during this decade.

The Tanzanian approach has to be interpreted against the background of the well-defined sociopolitical system. However, some of the innovative characteristics of the approach can be found in other developing countries with different sociopolitical systems. This approach is particularly attractive in that it emphasizes the minimization of cost of delivery of health services and therefore does not require great health resources. The Tanzanian example suggests that what is required is an objective examination of the health problems of the country, the definition of targets and programmes—as well as priorities—by means of a comprehensive planning process that adheres closely to the stated policy, the allocation of resources, and the implementation measures. The Tanzanians have attempted to ensure that their health expenditure is in accordance with the available resources. They are already looking ahead, as is shown by their involvement in a regional grouping consisting of eight countries in East, Central, and Southern Africa and established in 1972 with a secretariat at Arusha. Tanzania hopes to cooperate with the other countries on many aspects of health services so as to maximize the effect of their meagre resources and avoid the costly duplication of services requiring a great deal of capital.

The conviction is held in Tanzania that better coverage of the population with basic health services can be achieved through good policies, good leadership, and self-reliance. With a policy and a social system that place value on the health of all citizens, an advance can be made—despite limited resources—towards the better distribution of health services.

REFERENCES

1. Tanzania, Ministry of Economic Affairs and Development Planning. *United Republic of Tanzania 1967 population census*, Dar es Salaam, Bureau of Statistics, 1971.
2. Tanganyika National African Union. *The Arusha declaration and TANU's policy on socialism and self-reliance*, Dar es Salaam, 1967
3. King, M. G. In: *Team work for world health—Ciba symposium*, London, Churchill, 1970.
4. Nyerere, J. K. *Education for self-reliance*, Dar es Salaam, 1967.

5. Tanganyika, Medical Department. *Post-war development plan*, Dar es Salaam, 1947.
6. Pridie, E. *Report on the medical and health services of Tanganyika*, Medical Department, Dar es Salaam, 1949.
7. Tanganyika, Medical Department. *A draft plan for the development of medical services in Tanganyika with special reference to the period 1956–1961*, Dar es Salaam, 1956.
8. Titmuss, R. M. *The health services of Tanganyika*, London, Pitman, 1964.
9. Tanganyika, Medical Department. *Memorandum of medical policy*, Dar es Salaam, 1938.
10. Tanganyika National African Union. *The constitution of TANU*, Dar es Salaam, 1954.
11. Tanganyika African National Union. *TANU guidelines*, Dar es Salaam, 1971.
12. Rutman, G. L. *The economy of Tanganyika*, New York, Praeger, 1968.
13. WHO Expert Committee on Professional and Technical Education of Medical and Auxiliary Personnel. *The use and training of auxiliary personnel in medicine, nursing, midwifery and sanitation*, Geneva, World Health Organization (*Wld Hlth Org. techn. Rep. Ser.*, No. 212), 1961.
14. Gish, O. *Health manpower and the medical auxiliary*, London, Intermediate Technology Development Group, 1971.
15. Horn, J. In: *Team work for world health—Ciba symposium*, London, Churchill, 1970.
16. Reder, M. W. Some problems in the economics of hospitals. *American Economic Review*, **55**: 2 (1965).

168

"SIMPLIFIED MEDECINE"
IN THE VENEZUELAN HEALTH SERVICES

C. L. GONZALEZ [a]

In Venezuela, as in other developing countries, the provision of services to meet the elementary general health needs of remote and dispersed populations is a very difficult task. The problem has been the subject of growing concern and studies have been undertaken to find adequate solutions acceptable to health authorities, health workers, and health professional societies, as well as to populations. Such concern and studies eventually led to the development of a scheme known as the "Simplified Medicine Programme" (referred to below as "the Programme"), which has been gradually developed in the country over little more than a decade.

The Programme represents a long step forward in providing rural communities—especially those in remote and scattered areas and previously without any kind of service—with some elementary health care or attention. This endeavour relies on the use of peripheral health workers locally selected, carefully trained, and subject to continuous supervision. Although these workers are classified in the auxiliary category, the process of selection, training, and supervision provides them with the necessary skills to perform satisfactorily certain simple and clearly defined tasks of primary health care that can be delivered directly and continuously to people living in remote areas. Furthermore, these health workers are accomplishing their duties in a growing spirit of community service.

An attempt is made below to summarize the origins, conceptual basis, organizational and administrative features, progress, and present situation of the Programme.

Retrospective review

It is generally agreed that in Venezuela the modern public health movement started with the creation in 1936 of the Ministry of Health and Social Security (referred to below as "the Ministry"). During the ensuing period of little more than a quarter of a century (1936–1963) there were several

[a] In collaboration with I. Tabibzadeh, Division of Strengthening of Health Services, World Health Organization, Geneva, Switzerland.

events that deserve review, inasmuch as they led gradually to the implantation of the Programme. In fact, this review will help the reader to understand the reasons behind the proposals and the decisions leading to the use of "simplified medicine" as a feasible and acceptable approach to meet, within the existing conditions in the country, the hitherto unmet but urgent needs of people living in remote rural areas, for whom there was no hope of health care being provided by professional personnel. This period consisted of three successive stages, as described below.

1. The early situation

At the time of the Ministry's establishment, the country was under the impact of a number of communicable diseases and other problems such as a high infant and preschool mortality in both urban and rural areas. As has been the pattern in other developing countries, the Ministry began by developing specialized, vertical campaigns in rural areas for the control of certain diseases (malaria, yaws, leprosy, and ancylostomiasis) and also specific activities concentrated mostly in urban areas on tuberculosis, venereal diseases, and maternal and child health programmes. At the same time, the curative medical care work expanded gradually, although mostly in the cities. For small towns (about 5000 inhabitants or less) permanent centres, known since as *medicaturas rurales* and staffed with one physician, were created. The number of these establishments grew over the years, but not quickly enough, because of insufficient resources, both financial and manpower. For instance, their number increased from 71 in 1937 to 188 in 1945. A great effort was made during the following years with regard to *medicaturas rurales* and by 1950 there were 384, staffed by 418 doctors (some had 2 doctors on account of the size of the population). A study revealed that the *municipios* covered by these *medicaturas rurales* had an estimated population of 2.2 million, of whom only 800 000 lived in the towns, near the doctors. The remainder were people located in the rural sections of the municipios. In addition, 1 134 000 were living in *municipios* in which no *medicaturas rurales* had been established. It should be remembered that in 1950 the country's total population was 5.2 million, so an estimated 42% of the population had no immediate access to the services of a physician.

It was natural therefore that in view of the less privileged population's health needs and demands, the state (province) and municipal authorities (and sometimes the local communities themselves) started to establish a type of elementary unit known as a *dispensario rural* (rural dispensary). These were located in small villages and staffed by one usually very inadequately trained and supervised local person. In fact, this auxiliary received informal in-service training and was then assigned to a dispensary to perform a few activities such as first aid and to prepare for and attend the weekly or fortnightly outpatient clinic with the doctor coming from the nearest *medicatura rural*. The doctor had to "examine" an unusually large number of people in a short period (2–3 hours). The inevitable result was that the doctor's work had to be reduced to a too rapid interview and superficial examination (if any) of the patient, with no preventive or promotional activities, and there was no time for the supervision or education of the auxiliary.

Throughout a period of around 25 years (1936–1961) the situation was evolving. In 1961 the *medicaturas rurales* numbered 438, located in towns with a population of 1500–5000 people, and some 1032 rural dispensaries existed all over the country. In 1950 the existence of 482 of this type of dispensary was reported, which means that in the intervening period of 12 years 550 new establishments were created to meet the urgent demands of the rural population for at least some elementary health relief. In contrast, during the same period it had been possible for the Government to assign only some 50 physicians, to the new *medicaturas*. Unfortunately, these 1032 dispensaries were staffed by only one local worker (usually female) with very informal training and limited functions as described above. On the other hand, although these humble workers received little or no support, they showed human qualities, enthusiasm, ingenuity, and a great sense of responsibility.

Little analysis was needed to realize that this system was not viable since it was based on the erroneous supposition that a doctor located in the headtown of a rural county could provide general medical care to the entire population of the county, including people in remote areas. Furthermore, it was obviously neither possible nor advisable to multiply independent mobile units for specialized activities; what was needed was a staff capable of performing work embracing the main public health objectives, focusing on both the individual and his environment, for the people living in small, isolated villages—by that time one-third of the total Venezuelan population.

Indeed, before 1961 there had been some efforts to improve the performance of the rural dispensaries. The first recorded effort was made in 1948 in one of the states, where the regional health officer, after brief training of the auxiliaries in preventive and curative practices and in maternal and child care, initiated the delegation of certain medical actions to the auxiliaries on a trial basis. Subsequently, other public health officers made similar attempts, but, for one reason or another, all were ephemeral experiences.

2. The emerging notion of "simplified medicine"

The period 1960–1962 was of particular importance; during this time several events led to the adoption of the Programme, with the participation of a nucleus of high-level professionals in the Ministry under the dynamic guidance of one of the medical and public health leaders of Venezuela, Dr J. I. Baldó.

In 1960 Dr Baldó visited the Soviet Union to observe at first hand the modalities of rural medical care, particularly the use of the "feldsher", in order to be in a better position to prepare a paper (1) that he was invited to present at the Second Venezuelan Congress of Public Health held in Caracas in March 1961. In his paper, Dr Baldó suggested the use of a type of health worker along the lines of the "feldsher" but with certain adaptations to take into account Venezuelan conditions, which was accepted in principle for further studies.

The medical profession in Venezuela is represented in each major political unit of the country by a *Colegio de Médicos* and these bodies are grouped into the Venezuelan Medical Federation (referred to below as "the Federation"). As Dr Baldó's proposal was not well received by some of the *Colegios de Médicos*, it was considered preferable to experiment with it in a remote region, free from prejudice and criticism, where it was inconceivable that doctors could ever practise. A special trip was made to such a region (Territorio Federal Amazonas), selected because of the extreme conditions of population dispersal over a surface of 175 750 km²—almost 20% of the whole country. In 1961 this region had a population of only about 12 000 (including the estimated jungle indigenous population but excluding the nomads) and of 97 demographic aggregates only 9 had more than 200 inhabitants. Apart from the enormous land expanse and scarce resources of all kinds, communication presented tremendous difficulties; there were a number of rivers but they were badly utilized. The indigenous people suffered from extreme poverty and the cultural and anthropological characteristics of the nomadic or semi-nomadic population were still in the tribal phase. As a result of this visit a plan of action was presented to the Ministry, which authorized the Programme. It was in this plan that the term "simplified medicine" appeared for the first time. The experiment consisted of training 16 auxiliaries and then assigning them to a number of small villages where dispensaries had been set up for the purpose of the pilot project, together with the establishment of the necessary supervisory mechanism. The Official Report of the Ministry for 1962 stated: "In 1961 the experiment started in the Amazonas Territory. It appears that if the plan is extended and the requirements are met, it would be possible, with the support of organized medicine, to develop a scheme of *simplified medicine* in the rural environment, without having fears for this new system of medical care. There exists now the possibility of adapting controlling mechanisms which are sufficient basis to undertake new systems of medical attention, with simplified methods for providing services both in first aid and also in curative medicine" (6).

In September–December 1961 the author had the opportunity of observing the training and activities of health auxiliaries in various African and Asian countries. The results of these observations (*4*) were presented in February 1962 to the Venezuelan Society of Public Health, which recommended that a pilot project be undertaken to train a group of carefully selected individuals for rural health work.

It is only fair to state that the Federation had, since its inception, shown a great interest in the medical and health problems of the country. At its 1962 Assembly, during a discussion on the role of the doctor in land reform, the care provided by the rural dispensaries was qualified as "absolutely deficient and on occasions even harmful". Indeed, these remarks were valid inasmuch as the auxiliaries staffing the dispensaries had received little or no training, their functions being almost restricted to helping in the clinics held by a doctor who arrived after a difficult journey to stay only a few hours; in many instances the auxiliary was left alone because for various reasons the doctor did not come regularly.

It was evident that while for other auxiliaries, such as those working at hospitals, health centres, and rural medical posts, diverse training courses were operating, the numerous humble people working in the rural dispensaries had never received any attention, although a great proportion, even with little school instruction, had shown great human qualities and a sense of responsibility.

3. The Federation's acceptance of the Programme

All the events indicated above, together with the Federation's undeniable interest in the country's health problems, led it to consider the question as the main theme of its Assembly held at the end of 1963. For this purpose the group of professionals concerned in the Ministry was invited to prepare a paper (*2*) on the subject. The paper dealt with several questions, among them the demographic aspects, and included an analysis of population dispersal, an appraisal of health conditions in rural areas, and the scope and coverage of health services. It also developed the conceptual basis on which a practical and realistic but at the same time technically acceptable programme of care could be established to meet the basic health needs of such populations. Finally, it outlined the results of the field projects that had been operating for about two years on a trial basis.

It seems pertinent to summarize here the analysis made of the demographic characteristics and health conditions of rural Venezuela at that time, since it justified the proposal for some innovative approaches, including suggestions for substantial changes in the traditional system of health care delivery. The paper showed that of the 649 *municipios* in the country, more than one-third (233) were "strictly rural" in that none included localities with more than 1000 inhabitants, and 152 were "intermediate-rural", their largest localities having between 1000 and 2499 inhabitants. It was also shown that in only 126 (about 20%) of the

173

municipios the proportion of people living in urban areas was higher than 25%. These facts indicated that the problem of medical care in rural areas was not confined to certain states but concerned most of Venezuela.

It was emphasized that while, in proportional terms, the "rural and intermediate" population had been decreasing (to 68.7% and 35.7% in 1941 and 1961 respectively), in absolute terms there was an increment of some 174 000. This was of great administrative importance, since it showed that there was an increased population in need of certain basic services, including health services. [a]

The data from the 1961 census showed that 926 doctors would be needed in order to provide even one doctor in each locality of 500–4999 inhabitants, and 2373 additional doctors if one were to be assigned to each locality with 200–499 inhabitants. Even if this became possible, there were still one and a quarter million people outside these localities.

Some general indicators were used to show the health conditions of the rural areas, with the proviso that the crude data were not of the quality desired. It was shown, for instance, that in counties with more than 50% rural population, one in every three registered deaths was ascribed to "diarrhoea and dysentery" or to "acute respiratory diseases", most of them occurring in children aged less than two years. Other causes of death, such as tetanus, avitaminosis, and maternal conditions, showed a much higher rate in rural than in urban sectors. It was pointed out that, while the control of the first two causes mentioned above mainly rested upon an improvement of socioeconomic status requiring long-range programmes, it was necessary to look for methods aiming, at the very least, at decreasing early and excessive mortality.

The paper presented a similar picture of morbidity: the pattern was dominated by the same conditions (diarrhoeal and acute respiratory diseases) susceptible to therapeutic procedures, *the effectiveness of which does not lie in their technical complexity but in their application at the earliest possible time*, and by other nosological entities easily treated by simple, procedures amenable to standardization and thus applicable by auxiliary staff, given careful preparation and continuous supervision.

The paper insisted that the coverage of the population by the then existing health establishments could not be provided by mobile units, as it was essential to have a *direct* and *permanent* contact with the population.

It was pointed out that, according to the analysis made, in the conditions existing in the rural areas the real scope of a rural doctor in providing direct and timely care could not go beyond the town where he was located, and its immediate neighbouring areas (*municipios*). On the whole, it was estimated that only about one-third of the 3.5 million people living in

---

[a] Incidentally, the census of 1971 revealed that the proportion of rural–intermediate population decreased further to 24.5%, the absolute figure amounting to 2 632 000, which is practically equal to the one for 1950. So, in absolute terms, the problem remains essentially the same.

predominantly rural *municipios* had direct access to medical attention by professionals.

All this evidence, the paper concluded, indicated that a programme was urgently required which, in conformity with certain concepts and technical principles and with the financial and human resources of the country, would result in certain basic elements of medical care being brought closer to the people. This question concerned not only official health authorities but also the medical profession.

Since the paper was proposing a method aimed at bringing health services to the rural population, which had previously not been covered, the term "health penetration" was also used to describe the objectives. This had to be accomplished by reorienting the work of the dispensaries and integrating them into the network of regular health services so that they would serve as outposts of the rural doctor and provide, on the spot, certain minimal and well-defined medical care activities, both preventive and curative.

The paper presented to the Federation also included sections on principes and procedures for the execution of the Programme.

One of the outstanding milestones in the development of the Programme was the Federation's Assembly held in Barinas in September 1963, when the paper referred to above was presented and discussed at length. It is to the credit of the Venezuelan medical profession that the proposals were favourably received.

In the resolution adopted, the Assembly considered the proposal to be a "logical and nationalistic solution", reaffirmed the interest it had shown since its inception regarding the grave problem of medical and health care of the rural population, and supported the "Simplified Medicine Programme" as described in the paper. However, the Assembly called attention to the fact that the programme proposed could not be effectively implemented unless the principles and the technical and administrative methods clearly indicated in the paper were adhered to.

The favourable attitude of the Federation was also apparent at the Eighth Pan-American Socio-Medical Congress held in Montevideo in 1964, when the Federation suggested, and the Congress approved, that the experience of various countries (among them the "simplified medicine" of Venezuela) be used in areas where medical professionals were not available (*3*).

The Venezuelan health services

To show the position of the Programme within the national health system, the following section gives a brief description of the Venezuelan health organization, with particular emphasis on the different levels of the Ministry's operational units.

One problem in Venezuela has been the multiplicity of official organizations delivering health care (a recent study identified 84). Bodies such
as health institutions, medical schools, and high-level official agencies were
conscious of this situation and proposed to find solutions. It is of great
significance that the medical profession, through its highest representative
body (the Federation) formally expressed the same concern. Hence a
growing number of institutions and individuals are pressing for the creation
of a National Health Service to embrace all, or at least the most important,
institutions active at present. The studies necessary to implement this
new process were initiated at the technical level some years ago and it is
now to be considered at the highest government level.

**SCHEME OF A HEALTH DISTRICT
WITHIN A HEALTH REGION IN VENEZUELA**

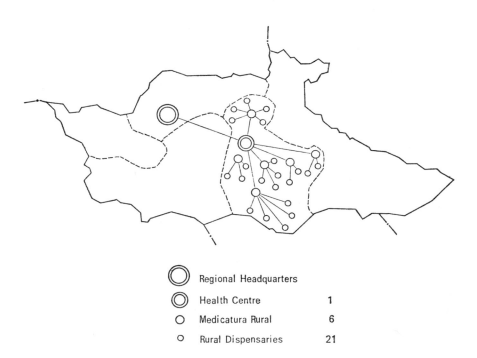

◎	Regional Headquarters	
◉	Health Centre	1
○	Medicatura Rural	6
○	Rural Dispensaries	21

While the idea of a single National Health Service was growing, there
was nevertheless a movement for merging efforts, both central (represented
by the Ministry) and peripheral (represented by the respective State Governments) in order to achieve some integration, through the development of

176

agencies known as "Health Regions" or "Cooperative Health Services". This step has been of crucial importance to the Programme, as will be indicated later.

Regional health services in Venezuela are organized on a common pattern. The service, under regional health commissioners appointed by the Ministry but also responsible to the state government, is divided into programmatic areas or health districts. The health district is the key element for the provision of general health care. Its focal point is the *health centre*, covering a population of 50 000–75 000, with a number of doctors (some specialized) and supplementary staff, with facilities for outpatient clinics, and provided with 50–100 beds for hospital care. Depending on the district's size and population, there are a number of *medicaturas rurales* (rural medical posts or subcentres) covering a population of 5000–15 000. They are staffed by one, sometimes two, doctors on a *permanent* basis, usually with facilities for outpatient general care, although in some there are a few beds, for emergencies, deliveries, and in some cases for temporary stays until the patient can be referred to another establishment at a higher level.

Finally, at the more peripheral level, there are the traditional *dispensaries* (rural health posts) located in small villages or towns with a population of usually not more than 1000 (rarely 2000); it is in these dispensaries that the "simplified medicine" concept was started and is being gradually implemented.

In Venezuela each regional health organization is regarded as a network comprising four levels (commonly known as *redes*, or strata). Thus, the regional centre, district health centre, *medicatura rural*, and dispensary are the first, second, third, and fourth levels (or *redes*) of the network, respectively. A typical example of this arrangement is shown on page 176.

From the above description, it is clear that the Programme, being a normal component of the health services, can be implemented only where there is an organized regional health service able to provide the necessary technical and administrative support. The Programme has had to wait until that requirement had been met and has therefore not been extended to all states of the country.

Programme development and implementation

Definition of terms

There are certain basic principles of a conceptual and operational nature that have directed the Programme since its inception and early phases and have remained unaltered. As mentioned above, these principles were explicitly described in the paper presented to the Venezuelan Medical Federation in 1963 and reaffirmed both in later publications and in the implementation of the programme. A review of those principles will follow, but it seems pertinent to explain the meaning in which the term "simplified medicine" is used because it implies the essential points of the programme.

The word "medicine" was taken in its broader sense, that is to say, with no restrictive connotation as to a special branch (preventive, curative, etc.) to indicate the comprehensiveness of the service to be provided, no matter how elementary it may be. The qualification "simplified" was added in order to indicate that it must consist of simple procedures of front-line medical care but having at the same time indispensable support in every aspect, particularly in technical advice, supervision, and referral to the higher level of the organized services. The difference, if any, is in the levels of technology and specialization of medical care but not in the existence of separate systems, one for the privileged urban populations and the other for the unprivileged rural populations.

Thus, "simplified medicine" can be defined as that part of the Venezuelan health organization with the specific goal of delivering certain basic health care through a cadre of auxiliaries working within a system that ensures continuous training, supervision, and referral.

Guiding principles

The Programme is built on certain fundamental conceptual elements, some of which are described below:

1. *Comprehensiveness of health care delivery*

No matter how simple the services provided by the dispensary, the goal is that the auxiliary should be concerned with the general health of the community and use all available resources to solve its problems within the norms and limitations established, referring unsolved problems to higher echelons. The important issue has been that he should not attempt, willingly or unwillingly, to replace a given specialized or specific vertical type of service.

2. *Continuity*

The health worker at this level must be available on a permanent basis to deliver simple services. The nature of the prevalent health problems and the essential educational character of the work are adequate supporting reasons. This principle can be more explicitly expressed by stating that: *"To be effective, any health service must be permanent. Diseases do not wait for the arrival of the health worker".*

3. *Supervision and referral*

The Programme presupposes certain delegations of authority and responsibility to personnel with very little in the way of formal education, involving, therefore, certain risks. Thus, it is imperative to ensure a system

178

of vigilance, in the proper sense of the word. In addition to administrative and technical evaluation, through simple but efficient reporting of activities, special emphasis must be placed on supervision and referral. Supervision must be frequent and productive both for stimulation and encouragement and for correction through education on the spot or retraining if necessary. The proper functioning of the referral system is vital, not only for the obvious reasons of offering the necessary care to the population but also to avoid frustration of the auxiliary and to prevent his being tempted to exceed the established limits of his activities.

Manpower and its training

The existence of an adequate structure for support, supervision, and referral is not guarantee enough for the kind of programme described here unless there is careful training of the key element, namely, the auxiliary.

Selection of auxiliaries

It was evident that the people already working in the dispensaries should be considered first as candidates for training, provided there was a reasonable assurance that their training was feasible. It was fair to accept this policy because most of them, as previously stated, already had some experience and, above all, a profound sense of duty. The candidate should be a native or resident of the village — a point of extreme importance. Since most candidates have only a few years of schooling, a minimum requirement is an ability to read and write and knowledge of the four basic arithmetic rules. Particular attention is paid to previous behaviour and the opinion of community leaders. All these elements, plus a personal interview, are the factors that decide whether or not the candidate is accepted.

The minimum requirements for candidates who have not previously worked in dispensaries are that they are native or long-term residents of the place, are acceptable to local leaders, and have had primary schooling of not less than 4 years. With regard to age, there is some flexibility (18–40 years), although the tendency is to take younger people.

By tradition, most of the former untrained auxiliaries in the dispensaries were women. In view of the dynamic character of the programme and the establishment of new dispensaries in very remote areas, it has been found necessary to train some male auxiliaries.

In addition to the auxiliaries employed by the organized health services of Venezuela, training is provided for individuals from other institutions, such as veterinary aids (Ministry of Agriculture), teachers (Ministry of Education), national guardsmen (Ministry of Defence), and missionaries of diverse denominations, to serve in very remote areas on a collaborative basis but subject to the same supervision.

The manual of instruction

It soon became obvious that a manual was essential, as simple as possible in regard both to knowledge and to language but containing the required subject matter, for later use as a reference book. The task of drawing up the manual was entrusted to a health professional with great experience in rural health work and in 1962 he produced in mimeographed form what is now regarded as the first edition of the manual. Since then, 6 mimeographed, limited editions have appeared, the last in 1968. This form was chosen so that corrected versions could easily be issued during the manual's trial period. In 1971 the Ministry, to celebrate its 35th anniversary, published the first printed edition (5).

Special attention was paid to eliminating technical terms from the manual as far as possible and replacing them with the native lexicon with the aim of both facilitating comprehension by the auxiliary and avoiding the use by him of language not understood by the local population.

Features of training

Usually 10, and never more than 12 candidates attend a 4-month training course held in district health centres (never in large regional hospitals, so as to avoid an environment too far removed from rural conditions).

The district health centre (or hospital) has the minimum facilities required for such training—outpatient clinics (both preventive and curative), inpatient services (for emergencies and common diseases), and a basic laboratory. Besides the district centre itself, one or two subcentres *(medicaturas rurales)* and dispensaries should be available for field practice.

As a rule, when the programme is to start in a given region a training station is established at the location of the health centre to provide boarding facilities for the trainees. Usually, a house in the town is rented for this purpose and is maintained by the trainees.

Originally, the training lasted for 3 months, but this was soon found to be too short. After some trials, a period of 4 months was adopted. Experience has shown that this is sufficient provided the course follows certain patterns, described below.

Firstly, it is essential to have a nurse specifically prepared and exclusively devoted to the direction of the course. It was clearly demonstrated in early attempts that nurses with service or other responsibilities in the centres could not provide the training. The nurse instructor is usually assisted by nurses from the Ministry's headquarters and by another nurse who is acquiring experience in order to become an instructor elsewhere. Other members of the health team (doctors, sanitary inspectors, etc.) help in the instruction but the main responsibility is with the nurse instructor. Experience has shown that doctors are not the best teachers for this type

180

of personnel because of their difficulty in adapting to the level of teaching and their tendency to use very technical terminology, which should not be taught to the trainees.

Secondly, the manual is the "bible" of the course, to guide in the teaching/learning process. Each part of the manual is read carefully and commented on by the group, with the help of the nurse instructor, who explains difficulties and answers questions put by trainees. Special emphasis is given to forming the habit of reading the manual on each case, understanding its content, and then practising, under supervision, the prescribed action, with either outpatients or inpatients.

Thirdly, great care is given to practical teaching. For example, the trainees learn to recognize the frequent, easily recognizable diseases (diarrhoea, pneumonia, malnutrition, etc.) through the presentation of actual cases in the clinic, without any theoretical teaching other than what is in the manual. The trainees are also given night duties at the health centre so that they learn certain elementary procedures for first aid in emergencies such as fractures, burns, wounds, etc., that require further care at a medical post, and how to treat minor cases.

As regards pregnancy and delivery, the trainees are not in attendance and are not supposed to replace the local midwives but to guide them in the prophylactic and hygienic aspects of their work, particularly in regard to what can and cannot be done. For this reason the trainees observe some deliveries with the nurse instructor, are informed of the main signs of abnormalities, learn to recognize the placenta, and learn simple techniques for preventing tetanus and ophthalmia neonatorum.

Particular insistence is placed on "learning by doing" in the case of immunization procedures, including tuberculin testing and the application of lyophilized BCG by scarification.

Finally, ethical aspects are stressed at every opportunity during the course. The instructors constantly remind the trainees of the confidential nature of all information obtained in dealing with a patient, the "human" approach to people seeking help at the dispensary, the absolute prohibition against using certain drugs, the limitations imposed on their work in view of their limited resources, the duty of referring appropriate cases to the higher levels of the service, and similar questions. In other words, as much attention is devoted to what the trainee should *not* do as to what he should do.

Services delivered

The Programme has been gradually absorbed as a regular activity of the Venezuelan health services. As mentioned before, a group of interested officers within the Ministry were in charge of its development at the beginning but gradually the responsibility became "institutionalized". At present, therefore, the normative aspects of the programme depend on the central level in the Ministry, while its execution is the responsibility of the regional health service concerned, for—as must be repeated—the Programme cannot exist in the absence of such a regional service.

The types of activity performed by the dispensaries incorporated into the Programme are, briefly, as follows.

Health promotion

Priority is given to certain elementary services in maternal and child health, environmental sanitation, and health education. For example, pregnancy is followed to detect easily recognizable danger signs that can be referred for medical attention; institutional deliveries of first pregnancies are encouraged; local midwives, who have been given additional training in health centres and are supervised by auxiliaries, are provided with essential material (kits) for attending deliveries, which must be reported in order that the auxiliary can offer basic health services to the child; children are followed up regularly for routine vaccinations, weight control, and supplementary feeding (skimmed milk) if signs of malnutrition are detected. In the field of environmental sanitation, very little is done except by means of educational and promotional activities that are developed in collaboration with community leaders and various organizations.

Health protection

Health protection consists mainly of the control of communicable diseases through vaccination. Auxiliaries can give the following vaccinations according to the norms established: smallpox, diphtheria–pertussis-tetanus, rabies, BCG, and typhoid. Polio and measles vaccines have also been given on some occasions. Auxiliaries participate in the detection of malaria cases by taking blood slides, which are sent to the malaria stations. They can also follow up patients undergoing medically prescribed chemotherapy for tuberculosis, perform tuberculin tests, and help in locating contacts and referring them to the appropriate centre. In certain states a tuberculosis case-finding programme ("rural bacilloscopy") is being carried out with very promising results. In these areas the auxiliaries, according to norms carefully drawn up, take sputum smears from suspected persons for microscopic examination at the district laboratory. (In some areas, there is a yield of about 2% of positive smears). Blood samples are also taken for syphilis investigation.

Health restoration

Health restoration is a major activity of the Programme. It is an innovative approach that brings closer, both in time and in place, some services to *meet* previously *unmet* but *felt* essential needs of people in remote areas. In fact, with the technical and financial resources currently available, it appears to be the only rational and practical way to obviate, at least partially, the deficit of medical care that was and is so evident in these areas. The approach consists of delegating to the auxiliary the performance of certain actions that in the past were prohibited in theory although sometimes practised.

The activities authorized under this item are regarded as "first medical aid", not only in what are usually known as emergencies (accidents) but

EXAMPLE OF A DISPENSARY'S MONTHLY REPORT

COOPERATIVE SERVICE OF PUBLIC HEALTH
PROGRAMME OF SIMPLIFIED MEDICINE

Monthly Report

To: *Medicatura Rural* of ....
From: *Dispensario Rural* of .... Month .... Year ....

1. Number of visits by the doctor to dispensary. . . . .
2. Number of persons examined by the doctor . . . .
3. "First aid" for diseases provided by the auxiliary . . . .
   (a) number of diarrhoeas . . . .
   (b) number of pneumonias . . . .
   (c) number of patients with stiffness-violet face *(mocezuello* ᵃ) . . . . .
4. "First aid" for accidents provided by the auxiliary . . . .
5. Number of patients referred to the Medicatura Rural . . . .
6. Number of injections applied . . . .
7. Number of dressings . . . .
8. Vaccinations:

BCG	....	Typhoid vaccine, 1st dose .
Triple (DPT), 1st dose . . .		Typhoid vaccine, 2nd dose .
Triple (DPT), 2nd dose . . .		Typhoid vaccine, 3rd dose .
Triple (DPT), 3rd dose. . . .		Typhoid vaccine, booster . .
Triple (DPT), booster		Tetanus toxoid, 1st dose . .
Poliovaccine, 1st dose		Tetanus toxoid, 2nd dose . .
Poliovaccine, 2nd dose . . .		Tetanus toxoid, 3rd dose . .
Poliovaccine, 3rd dose . . .		Tetanus toxoid, booster. . .
Smallpox, primary vaccination	....	Measles vaccine, single dose
Smallpox, revaccination . . .		

   PPD negative tests . . . .
   PPD positive tests . . . .
9. Number of births known: (a) live ....   (b) dead ....
10. Number of deaths occurred . . . .
11. Number of local midwives. . . . .
12. Number of local midwives under control . . . .
13. Number of meetings and talks with midwives . . . .
14. Number of pregnant women under control . . . .
15. Number of silver nitrate (or similar) eye-drops distributed . . . .
16. Number of umbilical dressings distributed . . . .
17. Number of home visits . . . .
18. Urine analysis, number of tests . . . .
19. Educative talks . . . .
20. Blood samples taken for serology (VDRL) . . . .
21. Number of tuberculosis cases under control . . . .
22. Number of samples taken for tuberculosis investigation . . . .
23. Number of slides for malaria taken . . . .
24. Number of latrines built with the auxiliary's influence . . . .
25. Number of children receiving PL (milk product for supplementary feeding)
26. Other activities . . . .

   ....
   ....

   Comments

   ....
   ....

                              ....(auxiliary's signature)

ᵃ Term for tetanus neonatorum in the vernacular language. Another term used is *mal de los siete días.*

183

also through the application of clearly specified, simple therapeutic actions for individuals suffering from diseases or symptoms that are prevalent, easily recognizable, and an important factor contributing to premature death in the community. Examples are diarrhoeal diseases and pneumonia.

Of course, it is vital to limit the auxiliary to this well-defined set of tasks. To this end, the manual that has served for training is used at the "bible" for the day-to-day work. The auxiliary is expected to consult the manual in every instance, to follow it exactly and not to take any step beyond the instructions, and never to perform anything from memory.

Referral is a very important part of the auxiliary's duties in the field of medical first aid and the procedures to follow in each case are clearly specified in the manual.

Miscellaneous

The auxiliary performs some other functions such as recording births and deaths in the dispensary's area (although it is not an official registration), notifying certain communicable diseases if suspected cases occur, and stimulating community development by collaborating with other community workers such as teachers, home demonstrators, agriculture extensionists, etc. Finally, the auxiliary is expected to take a "health census" of each family in the area, which includes basic data on the family and its members and on housing characteristics. The standard form for the monthly report that each dispensary must submit, reproduced on page 183, gives a general idea of its activities.

Other related programmes

The Programme has been implemented in Venezuela side by side with other related activities aiming at the overall development of rural areas. Among these activities the Rural Housing Programme and the Rural Water Supply Programme, also carried out by the Ministry, should be mentioned. Both operate in the same areas as "simplified medicine" and are coordinated by the regional health commissioner.

Administrative aspects

The dispensaries are mostly located in simple constructions specially built either by the state or by local communities. Although there is not a national model, in some states most of the buildings are of a similar type and include a section for the residence of the auxiliary.

The equipment includes some for the exclusive use of the doctor from the centre to which the dispensary is attached. He usually visits every week—in some places every two weeks for reasons of distance. The equipment for the auxiliary's work is quite simple and clearly identified for the purpose of each kit.

There are adequate facilities (refrigeration) for storing biological products and similar material. A sharp distinction is made between the drugs received for medical prescriptions (kept separately in the doctor's section) and those for the auxiliary's use, in accordance with a standard list (these include penicillin and sulfonamides).

So far, no vehicles have been assigned to the dispensaries, so home visiting or visits to neighbouring villages are carried out on foot or by whatever means are at the auxiliary's disposal.

All district health centres and most *medicaturas rurales* have ambulances that the auxiliary can request for the transportation of patients, using any means available in the village—such as telephone or messenger—to make the request to the relevant centre. In some areas, such as the remote places in the Amazonas Territory, use is made of radio communication, but this is exceptional.

The Programme is financed mainly from the normal budget of the regional health service since, as has been repeatedly stressed, dispensaries are integral components of such a service. Local communities help to meet some of the expenses—maintenance and minor repairs of buildings and similar requirements—but services, including the standard medication available in dispensaries, are provided free of charge to the individual.

Supervision

The insistence on supervision, a key element of the Programme, cannot be overemphasized. Even elaborate plans are likely to fail if this point is not adequately covered. Supervision of the auxiliary's work is carried out in several ways as described below.

During his periodic visits, the doctor in charge of the *medicatura rural* to which the dispensary is attached reviews the auxiliary's activities, indicates any failures, and suggests ways of correcting them. Experience has shown, however, that this is not enough for several reasons, among them the lack of interest on the part of some of the doctors, infrequent visits, and the excess of consultations. Therefore, it has been found indispensable to ensure a regular system of supervision by one or more regional supervisors of simplified medicine; they are based in the regional health office and devote their whole time to the supervision of a number of dispensaries. These supervisors are either former instructors or graduate nurses with additional preparation for this task. Experience has shown that it is preferable, even indispensable in certain regions, to use male nurse supervisors for this job. In fact, to accomplish his task adequately the supervisor must spend a great deal of time travelling long distances, sometimes by very uncomfortable means (rough roads, canoe, horseback, etc.). He stays in remote villages for a number of days in order to review the work fully and to correct the auxiliary's performance if necessary. When the situation calls for it, he may decide to send the auxiliary for a short period of additional training in an appropriate centre.

In view of the short initial period of training, this supervision is an indispensable component of the auxiliary's education. Thus the supervisor's approach is of the in-service training type; he observes the auxiliary on the spot, corrects his errors, and completes his instruction.

Progress of the Programme

The "simplified medicine" approach to meeting basic health needs of remote localities was not conceived and has not developed as a "crash" enterprise or a "vertical" operation, parallel with or independent from the rest of the Venezuelan health services. On the contrary, strict requirements were laid down before its adoption in given regions in the country. This explains the gradual way in which the Programme has expanded during its 12-year period of existence.

At the end of 1973 the Programme was operating in 12 of the 23 major political entities (states or territories) of the country. From 1962, when it started in Amazonas Territory, the progress has been: 2 states in 1963; 2 in 1964; 2 in 1965; 1 in 1969; 2 in 1970; 1 in 1971; and 2 in 1972. In these 12 entities only 315 of a total of 910 dispensaries were staffed with auxiliaries who had attended a training course. They covered an estimated population of some 280 000, so that an average of some 890 people were served by a dispensary. A great task therefore still lies ahead before these regions can be wholly covered by the Programme. As is to be expected, the progress differs from region to region, since the work started at different times and some health officers have been more active than others in implementing it. Again, by the end of 1973 in 4 of the states all, or almost all, dispensaries had trained auxiliaries, in 2 states about three-quarters had them, and in one state about one-half had them. The remaining 5 states were at various stages below that level.

By March 1974, 82 training courses had been completed by 836 trainees (an average of 10 per course), of whom 635 belong to the regular staff of regional health services and 201, regarded as voluntary, are from other institutions. In general, training stations for auxiliaries have been established in small towns where the district health centre is located.

It is extremely difficult to give even an approximate indication of the cost of the Programme; as it is a component of the overall scheme of general health services, no separate budgetary or financial accounts are maintained. What can be said is that the cost is moderate or even minimal if account is taken of the expenses incurred in other health activities and the cost of other public services. For instance, the direct *per capita* cost of training an auxiliary can be estimated at some 1800 bolivares (about $400), not including the trainee's salary, which is maintained. As regards the dispensary's operations, the auxiliary's salary is still relatively low in comparison with the pay of other workers, being on average 520 bolivares (about $120) per month, and the supplies and incidentals cost about 1000 bolivares (some $220) per month. In estimating costs, of course, supervision should be accounted for, both at regional and national level. Finally, account must also be taken of a number of indirect costs. However, costing is an arbitrary concept that should be interpreted in the light of each country's particular conditions.

One of the administrative problems is the high turnover rate of auxiliaries. As they are part of the regular staff of the organized health services, some move upwards to other positions. Others leave dispensary work on account of marriage, for family reasons, or because opportunities in other fields have better prospects. A follow-up of 595 auxiliaries trained and working in dispensaries during 1962–72 showed that about a quarter had left the service for one reason or another. The situation, of course, varies from region to region. In one of the states, for instance, the loss rate was very high (46% over 9 years—17% by resignation, 20% by promotion, and 9% by job transfer within the health service), but this particular state offers many attractive opportunities for alternative work.

A programme of this type is very difficult to evaluate in a statistical and numerical sense. In the rural areas of Venezuela there are many factors both in and outside the health sectors influencing the standard of living (and therefore contributing to changes in the so-called health indicators), so that it would be impossible to single out the separate role— favourable or unfavourable—played by the Programme. There are some indications that the Programme has contributed to the solution of certain problems such as tetanus neonatorum, which has been decreasing substantially and has even disappeared in the areas of the dispensaries. The increase in deliveries at the small maternity stations of the rural medical service is also an indication of the effect of the Programme.

But there has been no systematic, objective evaluation. Only recently this task was entrusted to the School of Public Health, Central University of Venezuela, with the support of the Canadian International Development Research Centre. This study is concentrating on the work of a number of dispensaries located in 4 regions that have been active for more than 6 years. According to the plan, the evaluation has been designed to inquire into 3 main points—the effectiveness of the services rendered, the community's reaction, and the cost of the programme. The final results will undoubtedly be of great importance, not only to Venezuela but to all countries concerned with the development of a scheme able to meet the health needs and demands of rural populations.

Perspectives of the Programme

Of course, in an epoch of such great, and even violent, technological and social change there is great reluctance to make predictions. Nevertheless, it does not seem too hazardous to state that "simplified medicine" has earned a definite place as a logical and promising approach towards satisfying some of the most pressing health needs of people living in the sparsely populated areas of Venezuela. In the basic proposals for the new integrated National Health Service of Venezuela, it is clearly stated that "simplified medicine", supported by the whole health system, will cover the primary health needs of the rural populations.

While the expansion of the Programme has been relatively slow in the past, there are reasons for believing that this expansion will continue more rapidly in the future. During the first 5-year period (1962–1966) 29 courses trained 269 individuals, 27 courses trained 249 individuals during 1967–1971, and during the two-and-a-half years from 1972 to mid-1974 318 individuals were trained in 26 courses. On the basis of the experience of the past decade, it can be expected that by 1980 the Programme will be operating, totally or partially, in all the regional health services. This will mean that about 2 new regions will be incorporated each year.

To implant the "simplified medicine" approach in each rural dispensary of each region requires considerable efforts, particularly in training. In fact, of the 1720 dispensaries currently operating in the whole country, about 1400 are not yet staffed with auxiliaries trained for "simplified medicine". Furthermore, this number will continue to grow as the needs and pressing demands of local communities are recognized.

There are certain long-range and short-range activities that should be undertaken with the aim of improving the Programme. For instance, the need to develop a special training school for supervisory nurses for the Programme has already been recognized. It has been suggested that a minimum requirement for candidates should be secondary schooling and that the training could be accomplished in 5 semesters, the last being devoted to practical training, particularly in treatment and emergency cases.

There is a need to improve the present situation at the "tertiary level" of the organization—the *medicatura rural*. This level is the "weak" element in the scheme, particularly because of the lack of adequate preparation of the doctors working at that level. In general, the doctors need to develop a more favourable attitude and better understanding of the principles and objectives of "simplified medicine", including the importance of a community-based and community-oriented approach. Some steps have already been taken in this direction.

Another long-range need is to explain the concept of "simplified medicine" at an early stage of medical education. Here too, efforts are already being made in several medical schools; during the teaching of community medicine, medical students are being brought into contact with the work of the rural dispensaries. Definite projects are also well advanced to arrange for final-year students to spend some weeks in villages and observe and work side by side with the auxiliary in order to get to know the real needs of the community and the ways in which it should be served.

Community participation and involvement are not very evident in the Simplified Medicine Programme of Venezuela, where an increasingly paternalistic and centralized form of government has developed over the years. No one would deny or minimize the paramount importance of educating and stimulating people to consider that an undertaking of this kind is something that belongs to their community. but it seems that education, although necessary, is not sufficient. A genuine community involvement in health or in any social development programme would seem to require profound economic reforms in the local communities so that they can become less dependent on subsidies from central sources. These reforms may need to be complemented by a better distribution of revenues so that the Government income is not so largely consumed within metropolitan areas.

Conclusions

"Simplified medicine", a term now widely used in Venezuela and increasingly accepted internationally, was conceived as a realistic, practical, unsophisticated approach to meet the basic needs and demands of people living in the most remote and isolated areas of the country. It is a relatively recent development, having been in operation for little more than a decade. Obviously, the "proof of time" is required before a final assessment of the Programme can be made. Nevertheless, the following points can be presented as lessons derived from the experience to date.

First, it has been shown that certain well-defined curative actions that traditionally had been, at least in theory, exclusively the physician's province can be delegated to auxiliary personnel located in remote and sparse communities where a medical professional cannot conceivably reside.

Secondly, so far no insurmountable harmful consequences have been observed—ethical, technical, or other. This is attributed to the great caution and care exercised during the training and supervision of auxiliaries and the well-defined range of activities that they are permitted to undertake.

Thirdly, there is a definite conviction in Venezuela that a scheme such as "simplified medicine" should not be implanted unless there exists a reasonable, regionalized structure of health services, offering the possibility of a two-way flow of communication for support, supervision, and referral. This is the main reason for the rather slow expansion of the Programme in Venezuela, but it can also be considered as the safety valve.

Fourthly, the proper selection, adequate training, and frequent education-oriented supervision of the auxiliary and his security of tenure are essential elements for the success of this approach.

Fifthly, it is axiomatic that the goal is to encourage local communities to play the most active role possible—in other words, to obtain community involvement. Experience has shown that this ideal cannot be achieved within a short time. On the contrary, it demands a great deal of perseverance and patient educational and promotional efforts, which will, however, achieve little effect if at the same time other elements of equal or greater importance than health care for the improvement of the overall status of those communities are lacking. These include changes in land tenure systems, improved housing, increased agricultural output, and tax reforms. In other words, no community involvement for health can be expected from communities in which the economic substratum is very small or even negligible.

In spite of all its limitations and shortcomings, and although an objective cost/effectiveness type of evaluation has not been made, it is generally accepted that the Programme has been successful. It is technically and administratively consolidated, supported by the Ministry's staff at the different echelons, and well accepted and used by people who otherwise would not have this resource within their reach.

To conclude, when problems result in the waste of human lives, firm actions are required. Health workers and society in general cannot look backwards and leave these problems unsolved. With this doctrine as a guide, the Simplified Medicine Programme of Venezuela was conceived and is progressing. Let us hope that it will be a complete success.

REFERENCES

1. Baldó, J. I. El problema de la medicina en el medio rural. *Rev. venez. Sanid.*, **26** (suppl. 4): 20 (1961)
2. Baldó, J. I. et al. *Estudio de los problemas sanitario-asistenciales de la población rural dispersa*, Caracas, Cuadernos de la Escuela de Salud Pública, 1966
3. VIII Congreso Medico-social Panamericano. Mesa Redonda No. 1: La medicina rural y los factores que condicionan su desarrollo, conclusiones. *Rev. Confed. méd. panamer.*, **13** (suppl.): 186 (1966)
4. González, C. L. *Impresiones sobre los problemas de salud en ciertas regiones del mundo*, Caracas, Sociedad venezolana de Salud Pública (Pub. No. 1), 1962
5. Lopez-Vidal, E. *Manual normativo para auxiliares de enfermería y otro personal voluntario*, Caracas, Ministerio de Sanidad y Asistencia Social, 1971
6. Venezuela, Ministerio de Sanidad y Asistencia Social. *Memoria y cuenta, 1962*, Caracas, 1963

HEALTH BY THE PEOPLE

KENNETH W. NEWELL [a]

There are few experiences as satisfying as success. But success can be judged in different ways; and what may be a success in one situation or through one person's eyes may be properly thought of as a failure elsewhere or by others. In this book ten groups of people have described what has happened in their areas or countries and all have described dramatic changes. Their starting points were different, the methods they used were not the same, and the end result varies. Yet all are successes. In this chapter, I have examined some of the goals, the methods, and the results in order to see if there were some general principles that could be used to help other countries and communities to improve their health. I am quite confident that there are and that we could be on the threshold of a new era.

My reaction on reading these accounts was one of excitement. Excitement that such victories in the health field have been won in many geographical regions, in countries with widely different political systems, and in some of the poorest rural populations of the world. By the use of well-accepted—almost conventional—simple health techniques and the provision of food, education, and assistance in improving productivity, the health of communities has improved dramatically and visibly and in a way that makes one optimistic about the potential for continuing change. *Technically* there is no reason why these countries should not have had the same success as those observed in Europe, the USSR, North America, and the temperate zones, all of which have also had large rural populations, difficulties of communication, and urban-rural inequalities. But, as one part of my mind tells me this, another part reminds me of the despair in looking at the developing world as a whole that was expressed in the introduction to this book. These successes, therefore, are of a very different type from those experienced by the temperate countries.

But excitement must be tempered with proper caution. While the reader is still glowing with enthusiasm about the possibilities for change and

---

[a] Director, Division of Strengthening of Health Services, World Health Organization, Geneva, Switzerland.

191

improvement, many of the authors quite gently but forcefully remind him that to really understand their achievements he must accept their goals. These are much wider than the conventional ones and range from that of health as a political and social right to that of health as an expression, or a spin-off, of a quietly functioning informed community. From this standpoint the authors place themselves apart from others who might judge success only by indices such as the infant mortality rate, disease prevalence, or the number of immunizations given. They do not question the fact that infants need food, pregnant mothers need to be delivered, immunizations are useful and prevent illness, or that sick people need treatment. On the contrary, they emphasize that these are some of the expressions of community action and that they will inevitably follow if you proceed in a reasonable way and take the wider issues into account. The wider issues presented include: productivity and sufficient resources to enable people to eat and be educated; a sense of community responsibility and involvement; a functioning community organization; self-sufficiency in all important matters and a reliance on outside resources only for emergencies; an understanding of the uniqueness of each community coupled with the individual and group pride and dignity associated with it; and, lastly, the feeling that people have of a true unity between their land, their work, and their household. With these as prerequisites, it is not necessary to bother to document the absurdities of the differing bureaucratic responses to agricultural, educational, health service, or development needs.

To some people, in the health field, such ideas may be strange, objectionable, or absurd. They could be said to be philosophical rather than practical. They could be thought of as an expression of arrogance because they are so all-embracing, while our backgrounds fit us only for "health". They may be more difficult to translate into action than the control of malaria or the provision of a water supply. A conscious effort is required to accept these ideas as essential qualities or to admit that without them there must be failure. It is easy to say that food is what is needed by a malnourished child and that community development is a mechanism that can be used to supply it. It is hard to say that community development is a goal and that communities in the process of developing find a way of seeing that children get food. These concepts are not the same. The way in which change is assisted and results are obtained may depend to a crucial extent upon which approach is adopted.

One can read the examples in this book in quite a different way and use them as a source of information on how primary health care has been delivered in some widely different situations. In such care there is a remarkable consistency throughout the studies. In all these societies, before the changes began, there was always *something* or *someone* dealing with primary health care. People helped the sick, babies continued to be delivered, and people obtained water whether there were formal organizations for the purpose or not. The indigenous or non-western health systems range from those in which the mother or mother-in-law assists during a woman's pregnancy, or a wise man or wise woman is asked by the sick for advice, to the long-established complexes of knowledge and experience typified by those in China and India. Some of these systems, while having their own strengths, may be fragmentary and ineffective in other respects, in terms of their effect on morbidity and mortality. A person can also receive western-type medical treatment in most societies if he or she has enough money, is willing to travel far enough, and is prepared to make the expected cultural adjustments. It needs to be emphasized that in all theex amples described in this book the new system of primary health care was either linked with the indigenous system or attempted to play a role having some of the same social qualities that the existing systems had. In this sense the new did not win over or destroy the old but achieved an adjustment that had some new qualities and techniques, and provided a link between the present and the past.

There are other similarities between the examples presented. Each country or area started with the formation, reinforcement, or recognition of a local community organization. This appeared to have five relevant functions. It laid down the priorities; it organized community action for problems that could not be resolved by individuals (e.g., water supply or basic sanitation); it "controlled" the primary health care service by selecting, appointing, or "legitimizing" the primary health worker; it assisted in financing services; and it linked health actions with wider community goals.

Another common element is the use of a primary health care worker who does not fit into the expected description of a doctor or a nurse. This person is frequently a villager selected by the community and trained locally for a period that could be as short as 3–4 months initially, an unpaid volunteer, or a person possibly partially or totally supported by the village people in cash or kind, and with responsibilities for aspects of promotional, preventive, or curative health. Author after author describes the primary health worker as one of the keys to success, not only on the grounds of cheapness but because he or she is accepted and can deal with many of the local problems better than anyone has done before and because he or she is *there*. The primary health care worker is no butterfly flitting in or out but is both present when wanted and still there to live with the results of his or her actions. You can also get rid of or replace him or her if you need to.

The relationship of the primary health worker to the remainder of the health services warrants a separate study. In some of these examples he or she is clearly a member of the community and not of the health services, as in China. In others, as in Iran, he or she is the peripheral

193

arm of the health service structure. In many of the others he or she has a dual role—community-based and community-controlled but also a health service member—and a clear intermediate link between the two. In all the examples the primary health worker is responsible for the mechanism governing the referrals to more specialized sources of help, and is the recipient of training, support, drugs, equipment, and ideas coming to the community.

There is no longer any doubt that a primary health worker of this type can work effectively and in an acceptable manner and that he or she does not need to be a nurse or a doctor as we at present know them. It might even be said that it is better that he or she should *not* have the type of training of such professionals. This in no way implies that doctors or nurses are anachronisms in other parts of the health services; rather, it emphasizes once again that the role of doctors and nurses should be re-examined and that a hard look should be taken at the selection and training of such expensive professionals. The difficulties of such a review are self-evident and, while urgent, such questions can possibly wait if it can be agreed that the primary health worker as described here can effectively be the main strength of a primary health care service.

In no example presented here is there a separation of the promotional, preventive, and curative health actions at the primary health care level. While this could be by chance or by biased selection of the examples, it does not appear to be so. In many western-type societies persons attending curative services are self-selected, while preventive and promotional services are often population-based. In a sense this could be said to be a historical accident as well as an expression of a system in which curative services may depend upon insurance or economic or social class, and the major emphasis is still upon the management of acute disease. But the spread of national insurance schemes or the widening of national health service coverage make nonsense of the first reason for the separation of preventive and curative services and the increasing proportional importance of risks requiring intervention at an early stage (whether this be hypertension, subnutrition, or obesity) makes equal nonsense of the second. If these are the dominating factors, the western-type separation would seem to be the anachronism and we should instead be asked to find reasons why there is a separation at all. None seem to be immediately convincing.

The "total health" approach does not in any way mean that all health actions need to be integrated in a single person at the village level. There are many cultural and other examples to show that in some societies actions concerning family planning or assistance during pregnancy, for instance, need to be dealt with by women whereas others are best carried out by men. There are other examples which emphasize that many villages are heterogeneous and that more than one primary health worker is needed to play a similar role in different parts of the same community. These are clear expressions of the need for a unique solution in different countries or communities. They are not arguments for separating preventive from curative services. Some of the authors in this book make the case that it is curative services that people want first (when health rises to near the top of their ranking priorities) and it is only later that preventive services are understood or requested. In this respect curative health services may be an entry point to, as well as a financial mechanism for gathering local support for, a more widely based programme. However, one can misinterpret such views. The examples here are all endeavours based upon *community*, rather than individual, health efforts to serve a local population. Individual payments may often be made for service, but the nature and the expression of the service are decided by the community collectively. The way in which this links curative to preventive care is well expressed in the example given by Dr Gunawan Nugroho. Here an insolvent self-insurance fund was saved by the consumer group understanding the reasons for an excess of the demand and was followed by community action on prevention. Many similar examples from China and other areas could be presented.

The arguments for linking curative, promotive, and preventive actions appear to be overwhelming, but those for a linkage between *financing* and service are not so clear. Dr Behrhorst emphasizes the need for a service to be self-sufficient by fee for service, but he accepts a new-style "Robin Hood principle" of differential payments according to wealth and discusses the financial links between health and the agricultural cooperatives. Dr Arole and Dr Gunawan use curative payments to subsidize a common health fund but also have common land or goat cooperatives as a source of funds or other resources. The Iranians use government money to pay primary health care workers, but some of the facilities and other contributions come from the community as a whole. While these observations are merely fragments of the total picture, they give one the impression that the financing of primary health care may not be a separate issue. Instead, it may be part of a complex that concerns the raising and use of resources for community development in the very widest sense.

The need for primary health care to be self-sufficient has been expressed many times and with a multiplicity of arguments. It has been said that there is not enough money in most countries to consider any other solution and that community priorities are more likely to be met if the people themselves both raise and spend the resources required. Such arguments can be valid only if the rural areas have enough resources, if the service costs are low enough, and if there is some source to meet the capital costs. None of the examples here have been presented in such a way that these factors can be properly assessed, although the assumption is that such services can be self-financing after a period of time, and when the development and capital costs have been found. In the national examples such as in China, Cuba, and Tanzania there was a re-allocation of resources for these purposes. In others there was an initial operating subsidy from outside sources and near self-sufficiency came in the relatively short period of 2, 3, or 5 years. But even in these examples the type and extent of the service were partly dependent upon the productivity of the area and the priority such a service had in the eyes of the community.

It is in relation to an issue such as financing that there is intellectual confusion; and politics, practicability, and technical decisions clash with each other without meaningful order. It is clearly absurd to discuss the financing of primary health care as a self-sufficient fiscal entity and as if any country has no health resources or other national health expenditures. Such a restricted view is reasonable only in so far as in some countries only a small proportion of the health resources are expended in villages. But if a widely based rural primary health care service was developed and proved to be largely locally financed, the moral, political, and other strains of having the poorest rural people paying for themselves and government expenditures being directed to the more privileged or to the urban population could well prove to be intolerable. There seem to be four interconnected solutions:

(1) to re-allocate health resources more equitably between all segments of the population;

(2) to introduce a programme of self-reliance and self-sufficiency to all segments of the population (urban as well as rural);

(3) to reserve a larger proportion of national health funds for the development and capital costs of the primary health care services;

(4) to redesign the existing government-supported (and other) health services to give them a more clearly defined supporting role in relation to the wide primary health care base.

The manner in which these steps can be taken is clearly a matter for countries themselves and one that should be consistent with their own image and their political heritage. In the Venezuelan example national resources were re-allocated for the simplified medicine programme and the clinics were redesigned as referral points. In Cuba the building programme was completely reversed and became rural rather than urban. In Niger a new supporting programme for the training of auxiliaries as the first referral point was given high national priority. National health convulsions such as these are clearly needed if primary health care in rural areas is to have any long-term meaning. Later I shall present some arguments as to which step comes first. Here, however, the point for emphasis is that even in a village (periphery) community scheme the link with national policies cannot be glossed over or ignored. The primary health care system cannot be thought of as only an appendage to an existing health service. If it is part of the day-to-day life of the majority of the population and is *theirs*, then it must eventually become the dog and not just the tail wagging behind.

Some of the examples presented here are clearly "successes", but they still must be interpreted with caution. They show that it is possible to introduce a primary health care system into a widely diverse series of communities, but they do not make the case that all communities are viable as communities. Some of these examples are from fringe populations on the sides of mountains or in the remote areas of otherwise potentially productive countries. An agricultural group that is landless or is made up of peasant farmers whose land has little or no topsoil or water will not become prosperous and self-sufficient in all respects even with organization and understanding. It is clear, from the long-term economic and development point of view, that some of these communities should not be where they are and that their land should be put to other uses such as pasture or forest. The studies do not show that by using these methods *any* community can be viable. In this sense none of these studies faces up to the primary question of social viability, which may be a national or international one. It has been asked whether it is possible to have a workable community organization and primary health care in a situation where the land tenure system is manifestly unjust or where the desert is advancing. The answer must be that it *is* possible, but that this may be just one step in a process that will eventually have to lead to a solution to the primary question. If one starts as has been described, it is possible that the solution will be found sooner, the possibilities will be clearer, and the methods used for resolution may be more likely to be evolutionary than cataclysmic.

All the people who have contributed to this book are doctors, even though their lives have been unusual and their present roles are different from those we normally expect to follow a conventional type of medical training. Possibly this is to be expected, and may be just one more expression of the control that the health professions have over the health industry. But as they describe their lives and their attempts to train and influence their colleagues and the nurses who work with them, one becomes aware of a bitter tone. None of them felt adequately trained or competent to undertake the work they found themselves doing, and few had access to many persons to whom they could explain their findings or whom they could encourage to undertake the same type of work. It is uncertain whether these leaders had a special role in health service development *because* they were health professionals. Perhaps their aura as a doctor or a nurse made them both acceptable to and trusted by the population and also an intermediary through whom people could speak to the administration. If doctors or nurses in many rural situations are not the right people by selection, training, or competence to undertake primary health care but could be its promoters, then it is likely that one must think of a different sort of health professional for this other role than we have at present. However, the case has not been made that health professionals *are* the best people to fill this other role. In the same way as the primary health care worker rather than the doctor or the nurse may prove to be the right person for primary health care, as being cheaper and more effective, it may be shown in practice that a new type of non-medical person may be trained and be the answer to the health service and manpower development problem.

Whatever the answer to this last unknown, it is clear that the health service education system will require a redesign rather than just a shake-up. What is required is much more fundamental than a new curriculum for the primary health care worker, a move of training institutions to the periphery, or an adapted community health doctor or nurse. If rural and community development is to be a series of progressive changes rather than a convulsive jump, the persons involved with health will also have to be able to change, improve, and adapt themselves in step with the community organization. It is possible to visualize a series of steps whereby a community could start by improving the service already there, then turn its attention to complementing it, and eventually reach a point where the service was consistent with people's needs and wishes. In such a progression many of the same persons would need to be involved at each stage, and their knowledge would need to change with the passage of time. One could not say that this or that amount of knowledge would be required for them to be licensed or qualified and that it could be fitted into a rigid educational mould; rather, one would need to evolve a way of feeding in ideas and techniques progressively as the need arose and the priorities changed. With this type of education it would be inconceivable that the present irrelevance of education to service could continue.

The examples presented in this book fall into three overlapping types:

1. National change (China, Cuba, Tanzania).
2. Extensions of the existing system (Iran, Niger, Venezuela).
3. Local community development (Guatemala, India, Indonesia).

Limitations of space have restricted the number of examples and it would have been equally valid to offer Bangladesh or Costa Rica as examples of countries that have radically extended their existing health systems by major national decisions, or some of the projects in Egypt or Thailand as examples of local community development with national backing. Despite this restriction there is absorbing material, which can be used to compare the advantages and disadvantages of each type of endeavour and to consider some of the characteristics that could be of use to other countries in following this path.

In the three national examples the starting point was a national political decision to change, made within a very wide frame. The decision did not relate to health only but included health among the rights of all individuals within the whole of society. In two of the examples the decision was also an integral part of an overall political ideology. The advantages of having the initial step be a political one were multiple, judged by health criteria and by economy in time. Even though these were poor countries, the clear statement of national decision and national will mobilized effort, gave recognition to health as something that was not imprisoned within the sectoral confines of a health ministry, and plucked health out of the directing hands of the health industry. Possibly too, a greater proportion of the national resources were put into health, although this is hard to document. The biggest benefit of this change appeared to be an increased ability to reorient resources quickly in direct relation to national goals, which in each case underlined the needs of the underserved rural populations. Each country came individually to a solution for primary health care which had potential even though its expression differed markedly from one country to another. The results were quickly visible, judged by the change in health status, and appeared to be most closely related to the primary health care system itself, to sanitation, and to nutrition. The changes in education for the health services, referral systems, and the supply and distribution of drugs came later and in some respects are not yet fully resolved. However, in all of the examples it was assumed that such changes would be required, and that they were a part of the medium- and long-term national goals.

In those countries that extended their existing health systems there were different goals and assumptions. In each case it was accepted that there were large populations underserved in respect to health, and that a national effort was required to provide them with services even if different delivery methods needed to be evolved to do this. Key persons in each country considered some of the alternative methods used elsewhere and then evolved a national, individual solution. There was no prior assumption that the application of this solution would be coupled with a change in the society itself or that the existing health services would need to be adapted also. It was even considered possible that the rural primary health care methods adopted might be temporary or interim ones, and that at some future time the country would be served by a single system with character- istics approaching those at present existing in the cities.

In the third group dealing with local community development, there was not only a difference in scale but also a difference in objective. None of the three projects put health services (in contradistinction to health) as the first priority and yet each leader entered his community with the intention of providing a direct health service. No decisions were made at the political or administrative level to change either the goals or the social order of the society, and all the project leaders appeared to feel that the development successes were completely consistent with and in support of the existing national goals. All three projects were separate from, but had an interface with, the government health services and with other sectors, and they were expected to have even greater links in the future. Their theme was that the new developments were what the people wanted, both in priorities and in the manner of delivery, and that even if other persons had tried to undertake a similar endeavour the result might have been very nearly the same, i.e., there was an inherent local logic in what was done.

These contrasting approaches must be a source of debate and speculation. The accounts do not include data by which it is possible to say that one way is quicker, cheaper, more effective, or more acceptable than another. All are successes when viewed from the projects themselves or from the standpoint of international objectives for health or because of the dramatic change achieved in health status. But these are not the only meaningful criteria; earlier I suggested that success might need to include an ability of most of the rural communities in a country to help themselves and to continue to evolve in an organized way with health as part of the overall development process.

If examined from this standpoint the third community development group presents few signs of replication even to neighbouring areas of the same country and the projects have not clearly influenced provincial or national policy. Yet all appear locally viable in the long term and all continue to change in accordance with their own development patterns. In answer to the criticism implied, it could be said that they were designed not to change countries but to solve local problems or to demonstrate new solutions to apparently insoluble situations within countries. I hope that their significance is greater than this, although the disillusionment with pilot projects that remain pilot projects is widespread. This innuendo can also be responded to by the argument that there has not been time for these projects to spread further. Weighing up these arguments and counter-arguments, I conclude that one of the ingredients in the success of these local solutions may have been the intimacy and intensity of the effort by the founders and leaders, and the fact that they were not designed with replication or national change in mind. A different sort of impetus and a different power base are required to change countries. If any country or the world is to profit from these innovations, the essential principles must be extracted example by example and adapted, so that they fit within a national context. Perhaps their weakness as a solution to the wider national problems is the assumption that if they can be made to work and be seen to work they will be adopted nationally. This assumption is at variance with experience in other parts of the world.

The second group of projects, which extended existing systems, also have their strengths and weaknesses. While they are clearly connected with the national scene and national decisions, their local strengths are less and their main thrust is more in relation to the health service and less towards rural development. They do not seem to be a link between local effort and a national political change but are a solution in themselves. They would appear to be of relevance to countries with widely differing political systems and to be a step that could be taken to expand a local effort to the provincial and later to the national level. The weaknesses are mainly the dangers of bureaucracy, lack of contact between sectors of government, and the reactionary forces within the health professions that could organize at this level of national endeavour to stop change. The Venezuelan account of these dangers and how they were faced is of particular importance.

The countries that started the process of national change by a political process have a clear advantage in speed and coherence. But the forces that influence such a change are quite outside a discussion of this type.

It can be concluded that in most countries health development as a part of rural development is possible if one goes about it in acceptable ways. These ways include the quick evolution of a village-based development organization and a primary health care system designed for that country coupled with a parallel national effort to build such a peripheral expression into the national scene.

This in no way means that all the answers are known, but it does mean that we have taken a step further and go on to a new level of questions, which include:

— How can the health and social development sectors be quickly adapted following national political change when and if it occurs?

— How can extensions of existing health services be adapted to become a part of wider developmental efforts?

— How can existing local community development efforts be replicated, extended, and made part of national thought and action?

— How can new local community development efforts be encouraged in other countries and areas?

— How can the demonstrated success of primary health care be presented to all who should find it relevant, including members of government and the health professions?

While the need for answers to such questions is clear, there appears to be no good reason why the world should wait for the answers to be prettily packaged and presented for inspection. There was a time when the problem seemed to be so insoluble that it might have been considered feckless for a country to start moving towards a novel solution. This does not seem to be the case now. The trail blazers have been out ahead and action that may have appeared in the past as unjustified has now changed and become almost a certain road to success. The "optimal solution", if such a thing ever existed, is not here but progressive courses of action towards an acceptable solution are with us.

Recently I was privileged to spend a day with a health assistant in a rural development project in Costa Rica. He explained his tasks of treating minor illness, supplementary feeding, immunization, family planning, basic sanitation, and health education. Finally I asked if I could see his records of births and deaths, especially deaths of children under one year of age. He produced his birth register but became embarrassed when he showed a blank sheet for infant deaths. "Children did die in the first year of my work here", he said, "but none have died in the second year. I have checked and cross-checked with the families and the babies are alive. I cannot account for it". This humble, successful health assistant was incredulous that his efforts could have brought about so dramatic an improvement.

It is possible that the world is now at a stage when it should no longer cause surprise that something can be done and that simple primary health care works. Health *by* the people may have come of age.

ACKNOWLEDGEMENTS

This publication owes a great deal to the Joint WHO/UNICEF Study of Alternative Approaches to Meeting Basic Health Needs of Populations in Developing Countries, which summarized the health care problems of the developing world and presented examples of some innovative health care delivery systems. The description and assessment of these systems were carried out with the assistance of the many public health experts who contributed to the study and of the teams who visited and reported on the projects, with the advice of a group of consultants who reviewed and assessed the findings, and with the assistance of the WHO and UNICEF staff who planned and implemented the study. All these contributions are gratefully acknowledged. Special thanks are also due to Mrs. E. Israël, Division of Strengthening of Health Services, World Health Organization, Geneva, for her invaluable assistance in the preparation of several chapters.

CONTRIBUTORS

DR MABELLE R. AROLE, of India, studied at the Madras University Christian Medical College, Vellore, India. After holding hospital posts in India she undertook a rotating internship in Cleveland, Ohio, USA, and then studied public health at the Johns Hopkins University School of Hygiene and Public Health. She is currently Associate Director of the Comprehensive Rural Health Project, Jamkhed, India.

DR R. S. AROLE, of India, is a graduate of Madras University Christian Medical College, Vellore, India. He worked for four years in a rural hospital in India before undertaking a surgical residency in Cleveland, Ohio, USA. Having studied public health at the Johns Hopkins University School of Hygiene and Public Health he returned to India and planned and developed the Comprehensive Rural Health Project, Jamkhed, of which he is presently Director.

MR MOHAMMAD ASSAR, of Iran, is Under-Secretary of State for Planning and Programmes in the Ministry of Health of that country. He studied chemical engineering at Teheran University and sanitary engineering at the School of Public Health of the University of North Carolina, USA. On his return to Iran, he was appointed Chief Sanitary Engineer to the Public Health Co-operative Organization in Teheran. From 1958 to 1960 he was WHO Adviser in Ethiopia and then returned again to Iran as Assistant Director-General of the Environmental Health Department of the Ministry of Health. He was promoted to Director-General in 1962, assuming his present post in 1967. Mr Assar is particularly interested in health planning and in environmental health; he is a member of the WHO Advisory Panel on Environmental Health and is Vice-President of the Iranian Public Health Association.

DR C. BEHRHORST, of the USA, studied liberal arts at the University of Kansas and at Washington University and is a graduate of the Washington University School of Medicine. For some years he was in general practice in Winfield, Kansas. In 1959 he moved to Guatemala and worked in the public health service there. In 1961 he became a member of the Faculty of Medical Sciences in the University of San Carlos of Guatemala. Since 1962 he has been Director of the Community Development Program in Chimaltenango.

204

DR W. K. CHAGULA, of Tanzania, is Minister for Economic Affairs and Development Planning in that country; he was formerly Minister for Water Development and Power. He studied at Makerere University College, Kampala, Uganda, and King's College, Cambridge, England. He was a Rockefeller Foundation Fellow in histochemistry at the University College of the West Indies, Jamaica, in 1961 and at Yale University School of Medicine, USA, in 1962. He has held academic posts in Uganda and Tanzania. He is President and Chairman of the East African Academy and Chairman of the Tanzania National Scientific Council.

MR IDRISSA ASSANE DJERMAKOYE, of Niger, trained as a nurse at Lille, France. After studying anaesthesia at the Aristide Le Dantec Hospital in Dakar, Senegal, he became an anaesthetist at the National Hospital, Niamey, and later medical assistant in charge of certain health areas in the interior of the country, including Tessaoua, where he cooperated with Dr Fournier in the training of village health teams. He is the author of a manual for village health workers in Niger. He is now in charge of Tillabéri Health Area, Niger.

DR ARNALDO F. TEJEIRO FERNANDEZ, of Cuba, a specialist in epidemiology, heads the research department of the national statistics division in the Cuban Ministry of Public Health and is Professor of Biostatistics in the Carlos J. Finlay School of Public Health, Havana. After graduating from the University of Havana, he spent some years in general practice in Cuba. Subsequently he was sub-director of public health and epidemiology in two provinces of Cuba and held academic posts in the School of Medicine of Santiago de Cuba, Oriente. He was formerly national director of the malaria eradication programme in Cuba.

DR GEORGES FOURNIER, of France, studied medicine and tropical medicine at the University of Bordeaux, France, and public health at the National School of Public Health, Rennes, France. An army doctor, he has been seconded to assist the Director of Health, Department of Maradi, Niger.

DR CARLOS LUIS GONZÁLEZ, of Venezuela, is a medical graduate of Central University, Caracas, and studied public health at Johns Hopkins University School of Hygiene and Public Health. He was for many years a member of the professional staff of the Ministry of Health and Social Welfare in his country and since retiring in 1971 has been the Ministry's Adviser Emeritus. He was formerly Deputy Director of the Pan American Health Organization. He has been concerned with various subjects related to medical education and public health, particularly rural health programmes and integrated health services.

DR ŽELIMIR JAKŠIĆ, of Yugoslavia, is Assistant Director of the Andrija Štampar School of Public Health, Medical Faculty, University of Zagreb, Yugoslavia, and is Associate Professor of Social Medicine at the School and Head of the Department of Public Health Administration. He studied medicine and social medicine in Zagreb. He is interested in epidemiology as applied to health care and the organization of health services, and in research in medical education. From 1972 to 1974 he was Medical Officer, Iran-WHO International Epidemiological Research Centre, and Team Leader (WHO) of the Health Services Development Research Project, Iran.

DR GUNAWAN NUGROHO, of Indonesia, studied medicine at the University of Sourabaya, Indonesia, public health at the School of Hygiene, University of Toronto, Canada, and nutrition at the Institute of Nutrition of Central America and Panama, Guatemala. His work has been mainly in the field of public health administration and research on new approaches to health care delivery in Central Java.

MRS RUTH SIDEL, of the USA, is a graduate of the Boston University School of Social Work. She has worked for several years with emotionally disturbed schoolchildren and most recently was Social Work Supervisor in the Comprehensive Child Care Project organized by the Albert Einstein College of Medicine, New York.

DR VICTOR W. SIDEL, of the USA, is Chairman of the Department of Social Medicine at Montefiore Hospital and Medical Center and Professor of Community Health at the Albert Einstein College of Medicine, New York. A graduate of Princeton University and Harvard Medical School, he has held academic posts in the field of preventive medicine. He has studied medical care delivery in Scandinavia, the United Kingdom, and the USSR. Together with his wife, Ruth Sidel, he visited the People's Republic of China as the guest of the Chinese Medical Association in September-October 1971 and September-October 1972.

DR ELEUTHER TARIMO, of Tanzania, is Director, Preventive Services, in the Tanzanian Ministry of Health and is responsible for the overall development and coordination of preventive programmes in the country. He studied medicine at the University College, Kampala, Uganda and undertook post-graduate studies at the Universities of London and Leeds, England. He has formerly worked as District and Regional Medical Officer in various parts of Tanzania.

DR K. N. UDUPA, of India, is Professor of Surgery and Director of the Institute of Medical Sciences at Banaras Hindu University, Varanasi, India. He studied at Banaras Hindu University and at the University of Michigan, USA. He was a Research Fellow at Harvard University, USA. He was Chairman of the Ayurvedic Research Evaluation Committee established by the Indian Ministry of Health.